Penis

Enlargement

Step by Step Penis Exercise Program

Enlarge Your Penis Naturally

Richard Nelson

Table of Contents

Introduction

The idea of being able to lengthen or enlarge your penis is something many of us are familiar with; whether it's through spam emails, jokes in films like Austin Powers, or talk in the locker room.

It's also something many of us have seriously thought about – whether our members are as big as they could be, how they stack up to others, and if it's actually possible to make your penis larger without destroying it.

This goal may not seem like an investment worthy of money or even time for lots of people, but for others there is huge personal and psychological advantage to having a larger penis.

The average penis length when erect (which is the length most of us care about) is reportedly 5 inches. This is, of course, the average and so is inflated by larger sized penises and then balanced out by shorter penises. In reality, most people have a slightly smaller penis than the average usually given.

Adult men with penises smaller than 2.5 inches when erect are considered to have 'micro penises,' with the potential for this size to cause long term health and functionality problems. Not just during lovemaking but also with urination and other penis function.

For these men a larger penis is a medical necessity, for others, however, simply being average sized or smaller may give them a feeling that they could be achieving more in the bedroom, or that they could have greater self-confidence generally if they had a larger penis.

Some models or certain types of actors may even have professional reasons for desiring a more imposing penis. There's no doubt that pornography has shaped how we think penises should look, but there's a reason people were drawn to pornography in the first place. It's the ideal many people have about sex and attraction.

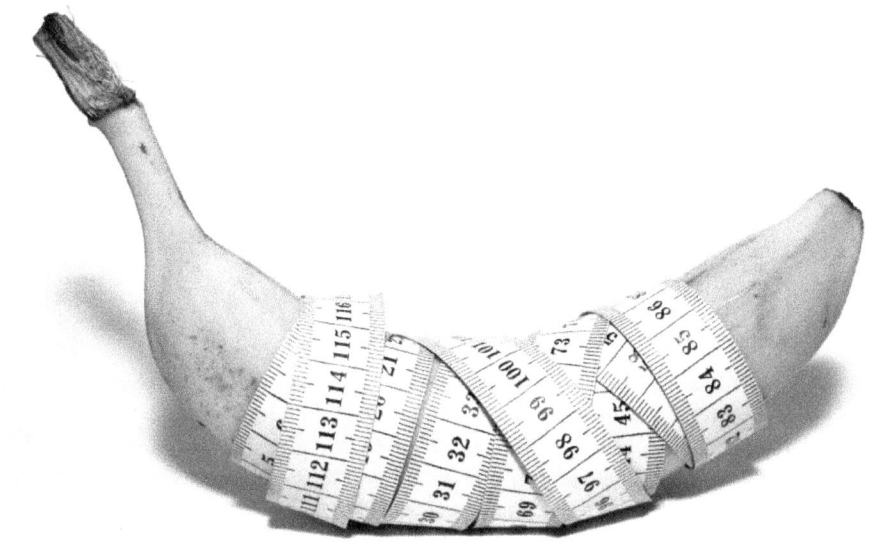

Is a larger penis a worthy goal?

If you think a larger member is of medical or professional importance to you, then it shouldn't take much convincing for you to try out the steps and techniques presented here. Yet most men looking for a larger penis will be doing so for cosmetic reasons and there is a risk that you feel such a goal isn't worthwhile.

Our society has a tendency to shame men for wanting to look better. Women may spend hours and hours learning how to apply make-up, getting their hair perfect, and keeping their skin soft and young-looking. If a man so much as thinks about going to the gym to get toned, however, he is considered vain.

Despite the fact that the biggest ladies men in the world take impeccable care of their appearance and physique, we're led to believe that caring about these things is not masculine.

The goal of penis enlarging is treated the same, but it should not be. The techniques and methods presented here are, for the most part, not costly or difficult to implement, and the value of a larger penis should not be overstated.

It's assumed a man's self-esteem and self-worth should be tied into his earning potential, but just like women, men need to feel attractive and to not feel shape about their physical appearance.

A larger penis may seem a trivial matter to some, but if the size of your penis is causing you regular worry then it's almost absurd to feel that way over something you can fix.

The idea many put out is that right now you are worried your penis is too small, but if you made it larger you'd simply find something else to feel bad about after that. The problem, so they say, is not your penis but something deeper. This is just not the case though, especially if you don't already worry about other parts of your body.

It really is possible that just a smaller penis is causing you undue stress, and, in fact, many men with these feelings report that they are far more comfortable with themselves long term once they enlarge their penis. They get a bigger penis, fewer worries, and far more self-confidence.

Typically you think of wanting a larger penis for the bedroom. A study by the Australian National University found that women preferred the look of slightly larger than average penises (though only slightly larger), so there's some merit to this. And having an increased size will possibly increase her pleasure, but will certainly make you feel sexier and more confident.

But this is just the tip of the penis enlargement iceberg, when something like this weighs down on your self-esteem it can slip into all areas of your life – from the boardroom to even approaching women for dates. Once you are stripped of this concern you can have an almost immediate boost to your self esteem.

How this guide will work

In the penis enlargement world there is a lot of misinformation going around and a lot of myths and strange ideas being presented as facts. In this guide we'll be giving you the information you need, based on actual research, so that you know how penis enlargement works and the options available to you.

We will start by looking at whether penis enlargement works (it does) and we'll try to give you a better understanding of your own body. Once you know how the penis works and how it can be made larger you'll be better equipped to debunk any bogus claims that come your way.

Then we will begin looking at the many options available - starting with supplements and medication and then looking into exercises, work outs, and natural or free ways of increasing your penis length and girth. You'll be given step-by-step instructions to ensure you're getting it right the entire time.

Next we will explore the various devices and gadgets on the market designed to grow, extend, and stretch your penis. Some are proven to work and some are bizarre contraptions designed to take your money. Lastly, we'll look at the surgical options which are open to you.

Where possible we will give you the explanation as to why these methods work and what is happening with your body when you do them. We'll finish with a cost-effective guide to getting a long penis without surgery, including a schedule and timeframe that you can follow.

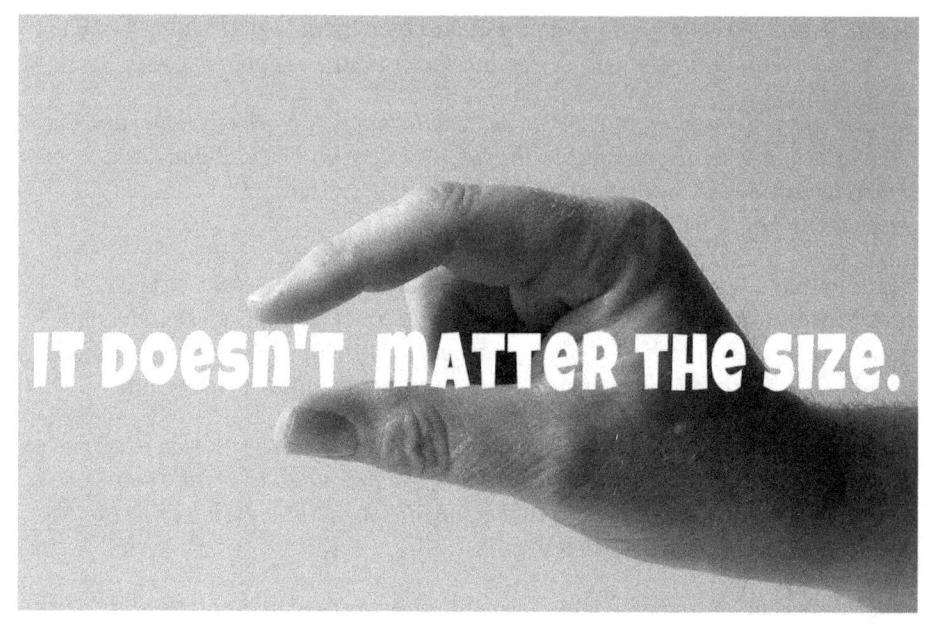

Is it possible to make your penis larger?

With all the myths and jokes surrounding penis enlargement as well as the huge snake-oil market surrounding it - it's important to start off by discussing whether penis enlargement is possible.

In short the answer is yes, and it's possible in a few ways, but first let's look at a few parallel examples of the body changing, so you can see how the human body is able to be lengthened in all sorts of ways.

Improving your body

If you take some time to think about it we actually improve and enlarge parts of our bodies all the time. This can happen naturally simply due to aging, it can happen due to exercise and physical correction, it can be due to medicine or diet, and it can be made to happen with surgery.

We'll explore these so you can put penis enlargement into context.

Using exercise and physical activity

One of the most common ways of using exercise to enlarge the body is with body building and working out. We take in extra calories and gain weight, then we tear apart our muscles with intense exercise and they grow back stronger and slightly larger than they were before by creating new protein fibers.

If we focus our work outs on specific parts of the body then we can have bigger arms, or bigger legs, or even bigger necks.

There other ways we can improve the appearance of our bodies with exercise. For example, while a good posture doesn't technically make us taller, it will certainly improve how tall we look - sometimes by a considerable amount.

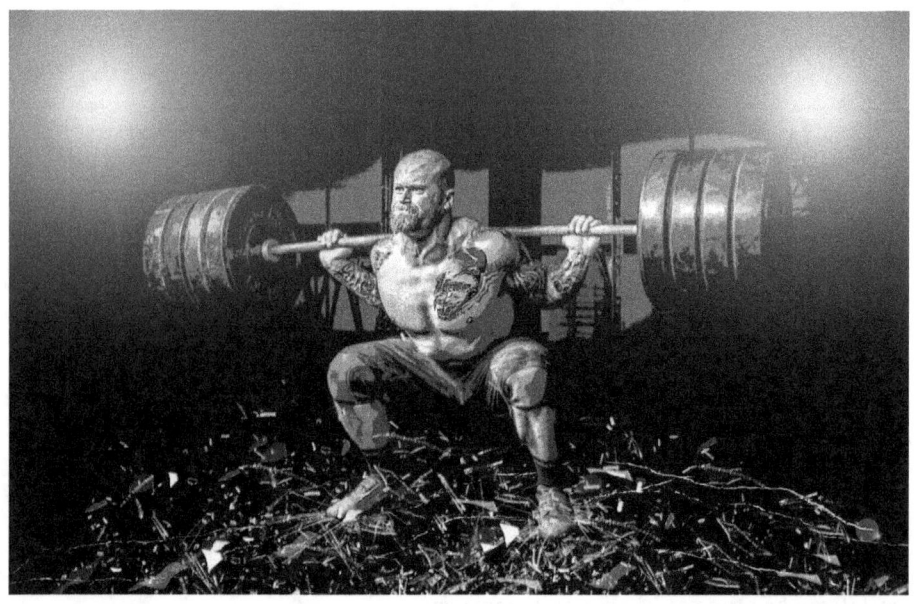

Simple exercises and certain sitting postures will force you to stand taller and gives a greater impression of height.

A study published in the British Medical Journal also showed that doing certain physiotherapy exercises regularly can make you grow by as much as two inches, as your muscles become more relaxed.

Not all parts of the body can be made larger as easily – trying to increase the length of your fingers is very difficult with exercise alone. However, there is also another method of increasing the size of some body parts, and that is stretching.

In certain parts of the world stretching parts of the face, including the nose and lips, has been a tradition for thousands of years, and more recently ear stretching has become a fad that can make your earlobes longer by several inches. Once stretched far enough they will not stretch back to their original shape.

So it's clear that exercising and stretching can make many parts of your body grow in length. It's true that this is not always growth in a true sense, but even if something just looks bigger that can be enough.

Using diet and medicine

Making a distinction between using substances to change your body and physical processes is difficult to do; ultimately all drugs and nutrition work with your body to create some change in you.

Again, here there are some fairly obvious examples of when we use foods and medicines to change our body shape. Steroids are a famous example – they really work to further stimulate the process of growing muscles that a workout does.

Androgen receptors are caused to increase their activity which releases protein building chemicals. The process is more complicated than that, but essentially it gets your body to reduce the time it needs to rest between workouts and encourages growth of muscle.

Famously human growth hormones (or HGH) are used by athletes to encourage cell growth and regeneration to help with the body building of exercise routines. Other hormones, particularly testosterone and estrogen, are used when people need to enhance physical sex-specific qualities such as development of breasts, a deepening voice, or the ability to grow bulkier muscles.

One of the treatments for people with a micro penis disorder is to give them extra testosterone during puberty. This is not to say that testosterone can be used to make your penis larger (overuse of testosterone can have serious health implications), but rather you can use hormones to make your body grow quicker.

Most drugs work by releasing some kind of hormone in your body so there is reason to believe other drugs could be used to increase the length of certain parts of your body – though there is nothing magical happening. It will have to rely on a process that exists in the body already that can be stimulated.

This means you can't take a pill that will let you grow a horn out of your head, nor do we have the ability to make certain parts of your body grow at will with precision hormones. But, if a hormone would make something like breasts grow then you can certainly take that hormone and accept the other things it will do to your body.

Our diets are also important, obviously you need lots of protein if you want to build muscle, but you can also increase bone density and help people to grow taller during childhood with nutrients like calcium and vitamin D.

Using surgery

Using surgery to change how you look is nearly always considered an extreme option, however, it is, once again, relatively common for people to change their appearance with surgery.

Implants in the face, buttocks, and breasts are common the world over, as is the sculpting of face shape and body fat. If you are particularly dedicated almost anything can be lengthened or shrunk with surgery – including making you taller by lengthening your legs. In that case the leg is broken in a few places and a telescopic rod is inserted to stretch out the cartilage of the legs day-by-day.

What to expect from penis enlargement

Hopefully you can now see that far from penis lengthening being an urban legend, it is actually possibly to change the shape of your body with a variety of methods – some intrusive and some perfectly reasonable.

Your expectations, nevertheless, should be set at a reasonable level to what you can achieve. Even with surgery you can only make your penis so much longer and adding several inches on is not realistic. Any adverts that suggest you can get a 9-inch penis is lying to you (unless you already have a exceptionally large penis).

The main methods for penis enlargement involve either muscle growth or stretching of the skin and penis tissue, and the level of growth you can expect permanently is not going to come to much more than 1 or 2 inches in most cases.

The average penis size

However, penis enlargement doesn't need enormous gains. As mentioned above as part of the Australian National University study, women do like the look of larger penises more – however only slightly larger penises. Surveys show women prefer penises of around 6 to 6.5 inches and they don't particularly like ones much larger.

A penis above 6.5 inches, it turns out, does not provide particularly much in the way of extra pleasure and if it gets too large it can be uncomfortable for some women. Not all women have the same sized lady parts, nor are they all able to achieve vaginal orgasm.

In a study done at King's College London only 5% of men actually have a penis over 6.3 inches long. Studies have also shown two other things, in the same London study 85% of women revealed they did not notice a huge difference between penis sizes and in a study done by UCLA it turned out that women nearly always overestimated the size of their lover's penis.

Many of these findings will be of little comfort if you have a smaller penis, but it does let you know that the modest gains you can make with penis enlargement are more than enough in many cases and women are likely to be more than satisfied, and most will even overestimate how big it is adding further length in other people's minds.

Welcome to your penis

We're going to have a crash course in your penis here so you can later understand why certain substances or exercises can help you penis extend in length in one way or another.

A penis comes in basically three parts. The root of the penis which is where it attaches to the body and in fact the penis is almost as long inside your body as it is outside (in terms of penis tissue). Then there is the body of the penis or the shaft, and the outer parts including the glans (head), and a foreskin. The skin on the underside of the penis is known as the frenulum.

Inside the penis you have lots of tissue. The two main columns that run either side of the penis (keeping the urethra in the middle) are known as the corpus cavernosum, which are full of blood vessels. The other large section of tissue that runs the length of the penis is known as the corpus spongoisum.

The urethra is the main show of the penis and it is a passage that pushes out semen and urine.

How does a penis get erect?

Despite being called a 'boner', the penis does not have a bone in it (as other mammals penises do) but instead relies on blood flow to become erect. When you become aroused the arteries (the corpus cavernosum) in the penis begin to relax and lots more blood flows in.

Once all the spongy tissue is filled with blood it stiffens and consequently restricts the veins in your penis that would carry the blood away. This pressure will let you hold an erection comfortably and safely until your mind leaves a state of arousal and stops the flow of blood into the penis tissue.

Erection Hardness Score

There is an infamous erection hardness scale which was created by the European Association of Urology (sometimes known as the EHS) that can be used as a reference for how hard an erection is.

There are four scores excluding 0, which is completely flaccid.

Level 1 is named 'tofu', and is the state when the penis has started to grow but is not yet hard.

Level 2 is named 'peeled banana', and is hard but not yet suitable for penetration.

Level 3 is named 'unpeeled banana', and is able to penetrate but has not yet achieved full hardness.

Level 4 is named 'cucumber', and is as firm and hard as an erect penis will naturally achieve.

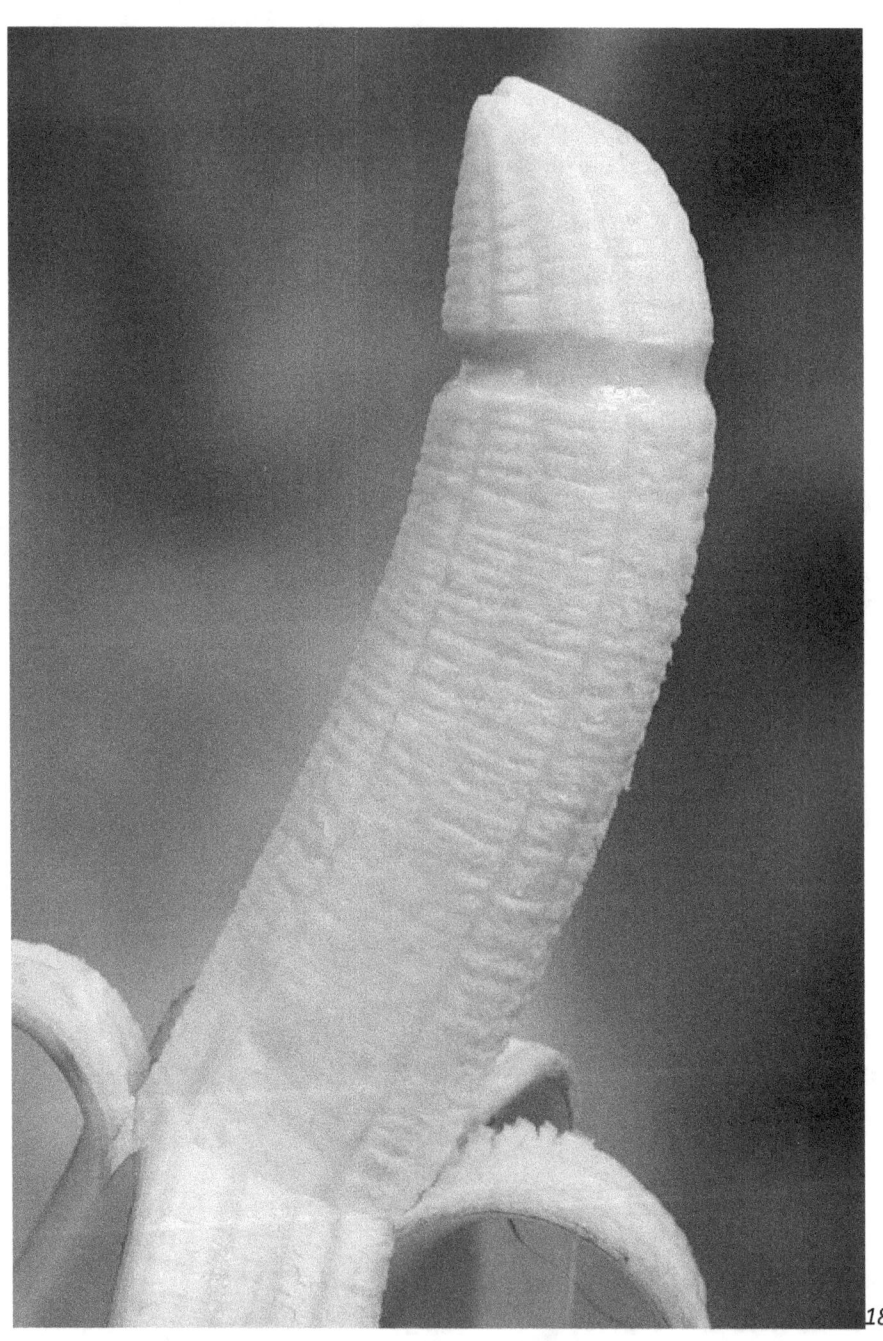

The scale is used mostly to assess erectile dysfunction and, while it's not as complex as the International Index of Erectile Function, it's useful because it allows people to easily describe the hardness of an erection. The names describe an analogues state of penis hardness.

This scale will be used here when the hardness level of your penis needs to be discussed. It's also useful to keep in mind when considering your penis size and it's quite possible that simply being able to attain a firmer erection could give you an adequate boost.

The relationship between a flaccid and erect penis

Contrary to what might seem logical, the size of a flaccid penis does not necessarily relate to how long a penis is when erect. A larger penis will usually mean a larger volume of penis tissue, but the amount of blood going in to make it erect is not necessarily more and there are no precise rules about how each man's erection manifests.

A man with a smaller than average penis may get a large amount of blood flow and pressure; he may also have a higher volume of penis tissue than another penis. You have likely noticed before that your own erections can seem smaller or larger, and harder or softer at different times.

Of course, this all makes sense because a flaccid penis can vary in size from moment to moment depending on temperature and other factors. This means erection size can also change and erection size doesn't necessarily relate to the current length of a flaccid penis.

This is all important to note as many penis lengthening techniques will make your flaccid penis longer, but that does not guarantee a much longer erect penis. If you have only stretched the skin of your penis it will likely roll back over the glans of your penis during an erection and some methods focus more on making sure you have a longer and harder erect penis.

Is a smaller penis caused by scar tissue due to over-masturbation?

It's no secret that penis enlargement is a field often run by quackery and one of the more bizarre claims out there is that masturbating too much throughout your life can cause scar tissue (or plaque) to build up on your penis.

This apparently scarred and mutilated penis, so the story goes, is not able to achieve a full erection because the chambers and erectile tissue of the penis are being constricted. Therefore you should use some skin healing balm to treat your penis and have the skin become more loose and pliable.

However, this is simply not true. Regular masturbation alone will not cause scarring on your penis and neither will any of the exercises mentioned in this guide. If you do have dry skin or scar tissue on your penis it may still be a good idea to moisturize or use skin healing cream.

There is a very real condition known as Peyronie's disease which can cause plaque to form inside the penis causing painful or weak erections, and in some cases an abnormal curvature in the penis (some curving is natural).

This is a condition often caused by blunt force trauma to the penis (though there are various causes) and if you are experiencing this your priority should not be penis enlargement, but a doctor's clinic.

A larger penis is not typically a solution to erectile dysfunction (thought it may help psychologically helpful), and you should ensure you have a healthy and pain-free penis before proceeding with any enlargement methods.

Making your penis look longer instantly

Before we get into the methods available for making your penis larger it should be mentioned that making your penis larger isn't the only goal you should have in mind.

Having a larger penis will not do as much for self-esteem if otherwise you still feel less than sexy; if you feel uncomfortable with your body in general then flopping out a slightly larger penis isn't going to cut it. If you want to improve yourself to feel sexier and half more self-confidence then also try to improve the rest of your physical appearance.

It's also the case that you can your penis appear much larger with some minor (or not so minor) changes to your appearance. If you're going for a larger penis you may as well go all the way and have the largest looking penis possible. After all, how big people think a penis looks is largely psychological.

There isn't any one thing you can do that will make your penis appear to be longer – it will require a combination of methods and body changing to get a really fantastic result. It's true that increasing your penis length can also boost your confidence and how you present yourself; however the opposite is also true, and how you present yourself can appear to boost your penis length.

Here are several techniques you can use to having a larger looking penis without doing anything to your penis.

Trimming or shaving pubic hair

There is a famous adage that shaving your pubic hair makes your penis look bigger and there is quite a lot of truth to it. This explains why so many men in porn have shaven pubic hair.

It's a simple optical illusion that is created without the crowding of pubic hair – but it is an effective one. Trimming your pubic hair can have a similar effect and many people find shaving their pubic hair is incredibly itchy and irritating.

Shaving can also cause in-grown hairs. If you want to avoid too much itching you should use a good razor, use plenty of skin friendly moisturizer, and use soaps and lotions that will reduce itching. After some time you will get more used to the feeling of being hair-free, however it never truly goes away and shaving regularly around the shaft can be difficult.

When trimming make sure the hair is dry and try to make an even cut using something like nail scissors. Some men like to do a little of both by shaving the hair at the base of the penis and on the testicle, but leaving some bush – this is known as the 'lion's mane'.

Exercising and losing weight

For some this will not be an easy way to getting a larger penis, however it's simple the case that a leaner body without a bulging stomach will make your penis look larger in comparison.

You do not need to be particularly svelte for this effect to work – you need only to lose some excess belly fat. While you are trying to increase the length of your penis you might consider cutting down on your calorie intake to gradually lose some weight.

So far there are not any real ways of targeting the fat just on your belly, but some small weight loss can make a large difference. Alternatively, you could opt to wear a shirt that works well for your figure and keep it on when you're getting your penis out.

Getting fit with exercise can be vital to improving your performance in the bedroom. Some types of erectile dysfunction are caused by a lack of blood flow and being more active can give you fuller erections as well as increase your libido.

Height and posture

There is not a huge correlation between height and penis length – but in people's minds there very much is a link, to the extent that a taller person may be viewed to have a larger penis simply because they are taller.

Tied into this is the perception that tall people are more confident and, for some reason, we tie penis length into confidence and masculinity. Our ideas about the world can actually change how we perceive it – most famously when lazy people guess distances to be further away than active people do.

What this means is that if you can do things to make yourself exude confidence and appear taller, then people will perceive your penis to be larger – both when you are clothed and unclothed.

Your posture is vital in appearing as tall as possible and it is also generally important when wondering about the imposingness of your penis. If you arch your back and bend over you are necessarily hiding your penis away and making it appear shorter. Improving your posture is, therefore, an important step to having a penis that will thrust out and appear more bulky.

Foreplay and sexual arousal

As mentioned earlier, getting an erection starts off in your mind. It's primarily a psychological phenomenon and the more aroused you are the longer you can maintain an erection and the fuller it will be.

Only so much blood can flow into your penis during an erection, but the stronger your arousal states are stimulated the more blood your body will send to it. The only thing keeping your erection in place is your state of arousal and no doubt you've experienced soft erections when you were only half aroused before. Equally then, you can produce much harder erections if you will it.

What this all means is that if you want a guaranteed longer erection all you need do is become more aroused and to have more intense erotic situations. There are many ways you can do this and largely it is up to personal preference; however, things you may want to try include longer foreplay *sessions (where the focus for you is becoming sexually excited – not just priming your partner for sex), trying out novel sexual situations (exploring fetishes, new positions, different clothes etc.), and really taking you time with lovemaking (avoiding the perfunctory quickie).*

On the other end of the spectrum are the things stopping you getting a full erection. One of the most well known issues is the infamous 'whisky dick' that men experience after drinking too much.

More commonly some men experience anxiety, especially if they are self conscious about the size of their penis, or if they are inexperienced, or with a new sexual partner. Relaxation is an important part of arousal and so you want to make sure you are as comfortable as possible when trying to get an erection. Foreplay, again, can be a solution here as it often reduces awkwardness and anxiety.

Controlling your environment

Lastly, and one of the easiest points here, is controlling your environment. This can be surprisingly effective for having both a longer flaccid and erect penis.

The simple fact is that if you're feeling cold and on edge your penis will be smaller. Making sure you are in a warm room, giving yourself extra privacy, and being well hydrated can all contribute to a temporarily longer penis.

You can help this further along by doing something such as taking a long hot bath.

Cock ring

On many supermarket shelves you'll find cock rings beings sold next to condoms, and they are a staple item in sex shops around the world. They come in a large variety of shapes and materials. Some are triple-looped metal devices, made to go around your testicles, and others have vibrating elements to stimulate a clitoris during sex.

Many of these are clearly fetish items with their own unique thrills, but the basic purpose is to trap blood inside your penis so that you can hold an erection for longer, while making sure it's fuller and also highlights the veins along the shaft.

Later we will look at the use of clamps for penis enlargement, but you might want to consider a cock ring for a quick and easy way to get more imposing penis. They won't really make it any bigger, but it can be psychology exciting, and you should have a noticeably fuller erection for longer.

Penis extender sleeve

In sex shops you will find two types of penis extender. One is a device for stretching the penis out (more on them later), and the other is a sleeve that you can slip on over your penis to extend its length and girth.

Once again, in many instances these are a fetish item and for most men they will not address the real concerns about penis length. In addition, they will inhibit pleasure and may not function as well as they might appear to.

However, these should be mentioned as an option because in some instances they may be the ideal solution and they are quick, easy, and cheap to get. For example, if you just have a fetish for larger penises, or you are particularly considered about pleasuring a woman with a longer penis.

Staying safe and having a longer penis

All of the methods and techniques suggested in this book are safe and can be done by most people of reasonable health. However, a small warning should be made here as some people may get impatient and overload themselves with pills, stretching, and exercises leading to a real possibility of harm.

If a stretching method, for example, says not to stretch too much in a day do not try to do double for more effective or quicker results. Penis enlargement is best done with small gains over a long period of time.

If you have issues with blood pressure or a heart condition then take extra caution when using any medication or pressure-based penis enlargement as it may have some unintended side effects for you.

When taking on a new exercise routine or dealing with a sensitive part of your body begin gently and make sure you are comfortable with what you are doing before you take it further.

Exercise routines

By far the cheapest and simplest way to increase your penis length is with daily exercise. Here you will be focusing on working out your penis, stretching your penis tissue, and improving the muscle strength of your pelvis and genital areas.

These techniques are often overlooked in the penis enlargement world because they don't guarantee instant results, it's harder to make money off them, and the gains you can make doing this are modest.

Nevertheless, these are techniques that have been tested and proven, and men the world over use them in their daily routines. Not only will some of these exercises increase penis length and girth, but they can also help you have greater control over your penis. This means you have better power to prevent urine leakages and to hold back ejaculation during sex.

We'll start by looking at how the techniques work and then consider ways you could include them in a daily workout routine.

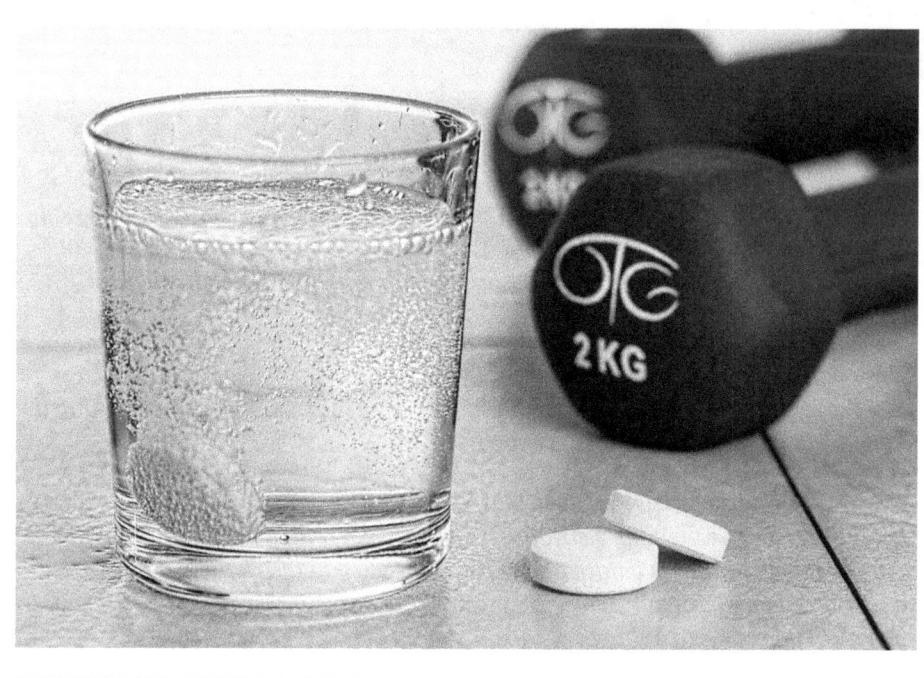

Basic penis warm-ups

Penis exercises are like any other type of workout and the best and safest results will always come if you do some warming up. You're not risking any real injury without warming-up for most of the exercises here, but when working out a routine it's good to have some of these techniques mastered.

Here we'll list some of the most successful routines that can be easily incorporated into your chosen work-out.

Hot towel warm-up

This is a literal warm-up and besides feeling good it really loosens up your penis so that it is pliable and easy to work with.

1. Soak a towel (or similar) in warm water (warm enough to really feel the heat but not burn your body). Ensure it is not too saturated by wringing it out once soaked.

2. Cover your penis, testicles, and general groin area with the towel and keep enveloped for a minute.

3. Repeat the warm-up once or twice more and re-heat the towel as necessary.

You could also use a heating pad or rice sock for a similar effect or you may choose to have a warm bath or hot shower. Several of the penis lengthening exercises benefit from being done in a warm and wet environment like the bath or shower anyway.

Some choose to use an infrared lamp, but that is largely unnecessary to get the required warmth and relaxation.

Inchworm warm-up

The inch worm is a well loved warm-up exercise that is great for getting your pelvis region feeling limber and ready for a heavier dynamic workout. This is called the inchworm because you will move forward and go up and down the way that a worm or caterpillar does.

1. Begin by standing and then bend and touch the floor with your fingers while you keep your legs straight – this should cause some stretching in your hamstrings.

2. While keeping your feet in place walk your arms forwards until you are in a position where you could do a push-up – keep as straight as possible while here.

3. Keeping your arms in place begin to walk you feet up towards where your hands are (though you don't need to get too close) while keeping your legs straight. Your buttocks and hips will be raised in the air while you do this.

4. With your feet near your hands, perform an action similar to step two where your walk your hands forwards until you are in a push-up position.

5. Repeat this at least six times and try to give yourself a good stretch without straining your back.

Thigh Stretch

This is another classic and simple stretch that will get your thighs feeling loose and can get your lower feeling taught and more in control. In short all you need to do is bend each leg while facing forwards.

1. Begin by standing up and then bend your right knee back using one arm. Don't do this quickly and try to bend your knee as far back as it will go – pull your foot so that it's as level as possible.

 For this to work without you falling over it's a good idea to have a low surface or wall to lean against with your other hand.

2. Bend forward until your torso and bent leg are parallel to the ground. This should require a stretch in your thighs and hamstrings.

Pelvic Curl

The pelvic curl is a staple stretch for Pilates and it works well here to prime your pelvis area for further exercise. For many penis exercises the warm-ups may be as intense as the exercise, but they're still useful for getting active and getting in the right mind-set.

1. Begin by lying down on the floor with your head facing up, your knees bent, and your arms either side of you on the floor – palms facing down.

2. With your arms in place and your head and feet still touching the floor move your pelvis and lower back up into the air. Keep a straight line with your body and hold for at least 5 seconds.

3. Lower your body to the position in step 1 and then repeat at least 15 times.

Simple stretch exercises

Not all exercises for your penis need be difficult or done as part of a rigorous routine. You can also do some lighter stretches that can be used during your daily activities, or when sat around watching television. It's easier to do this with stretching as it doesn't require an erection, lubricant, or much strain.

The only caveat is that you should try to be as hygienic as possible when doing this; however, many people have a frankly odd idea of the kind of bacteria that will be located on a recently cleaned penis. Making sure you keep your hands clean before eating should be more than sufficient.

Avoid stretching for too long or with too much force. Keep these things to a maximum of one hour a day, but don't be afraid to try them daily as they can be powerful aids in enlarging your penis.

Basic Penis Stretch

This is an extremely simple stretch and can be used for a quick 2 to 5 minutes warm-up before you begin your other exercises or techniques. The fact that it is so simple, however, means the gains you'll get from it alone will not be too effective.

1. Grab your penis firmly, but not with too much pressure, just below the glans.

2. Pull your penis either right, left, upwards, downwards, or straight out as far as you comfortably can.

Sit and Stretch

This is a very simple stretch, that some will even find pleasurable. The effects of it are not going to be profound but it can help compound other stretching efforts.

1. Warm your penis up until it lengthens but don't quite go to a level 2 erection.

2. Tuck your penis between your legs, underneath the fat part of your thighs, and then sit down on a flat chair or surface. You should feel some pressure on your penis here, but it should not be painful.

3. Sit for at least 20 minutes like this and if you feel you are going too flaccid, don't be afraid to re-work your penis into a semi-erect state.

Jelqing

'Jelqing' has been a big thing in the penis enlargement community for a long time and with good reason. If you've explored penis enlargement at all, then it's likely you've already heard about it.

In short jelqing is a simple exercise where the penis is 'milked' for several minutes a day to increase circulation and allow for more blood to flow to your penis during an erection, as well as a general strengthening of the penis.

A jelq is quite different to simply stroking the penis for a few minutes – you're not just jerking off. You need to do it in a concerted way and to give your member a legitimate work-out.

Gains can be slow here, but when done consistently and used in effect with other methods, people have reported consistent gains of 1 to 2 inches of penis length. The key, of course, being the consistency of the jelqing – just as you wouldn't expect massive arms from only a few minutes of weight lifting every so often, don't expect a longer penis without commitment.

With that said the penis itself does not have any technical muscles (though specific muscles can be grown to support the penis), so a regular physical workout will not necessarily do much to increase penis size. Instead the physical exercise has to either stretch the skin of penis, or increase its capacity for storing blood by expanding the size of the erectile tissue.

Jelqing aims to do the latter so you will be able to have more volume in general and a longer and firmer erection. This is done by trying to stretch the penis tissue for a sustained period of time each day – both while flaccid and semi-

erect. The larger the tissue is in the penis, the more room there is to store hot blood.

What kind of results can I expect?

'Jelqing', as the name implies when you said it aloud, comes from an old Arabic word meaning 'milking', and it's from that ancient tradition that its gets its footing. Proper clinical research has not yet been done on the technique, but the popularity of it and the huge volumes of testimony and evidence, suggest that it is relatively effective.

General reports indicate that you can expect to start seeing growth after one month, with some people taking up to three or four months to see measurable results. From then on growths of three inches have been consistently reported among many people.

This time frame is as much a reflection of people as the technique itself. Effective jelqing requires a holistic approach of better fitness and people report much better results when jelqing is used as part of a more intense body workout.

After the gains seen in the first 6 months you may have to use more intense jelqing to see addition gains – which could lead to injury. It's best to accept a more modest gain that you can be truly happy and comfortable with.

Increases in length made with jelqing should be permanent, but as with any stretching of the body it will naturally return closer to its original state without at least some regular jelqing sessions. Nevertheless, you will not need to carry our 10 minute jelqing sessions forever.

The additional bonus of practicing jelqing is that you will become much better at achieving a full erection and knowing how to sustain it.

Given the nature of the exercise, as you'll see next, this exercise mostly increases the length of the penis and not the girth. A regime that increases both girth and length will need to incorporate different exercises or combine jelqing with other techniques or supplements.

To begin you will want to lubricate your penis so you can create a nice sliding sensation and you can give your whole penis shaft a workout. You do not need any heavy duty lubricant for this as getting started with a good flow should be enough.

Water alone will not help stop too much friction, but you may be able to make do with saliva or high-lather skin-friendly shampoo. If you want more substance then something such as baby oil should be fine – expensive sexual lubricants are generally unnecessary and the price will add up if used too every day.

Avoid any lubricants that are sugar based as, despites some myths, men are also able to get a rash when this contacts sensitive parts of their penis. Dry jelqing can be unpleasant and could create a rash also if done persistently.

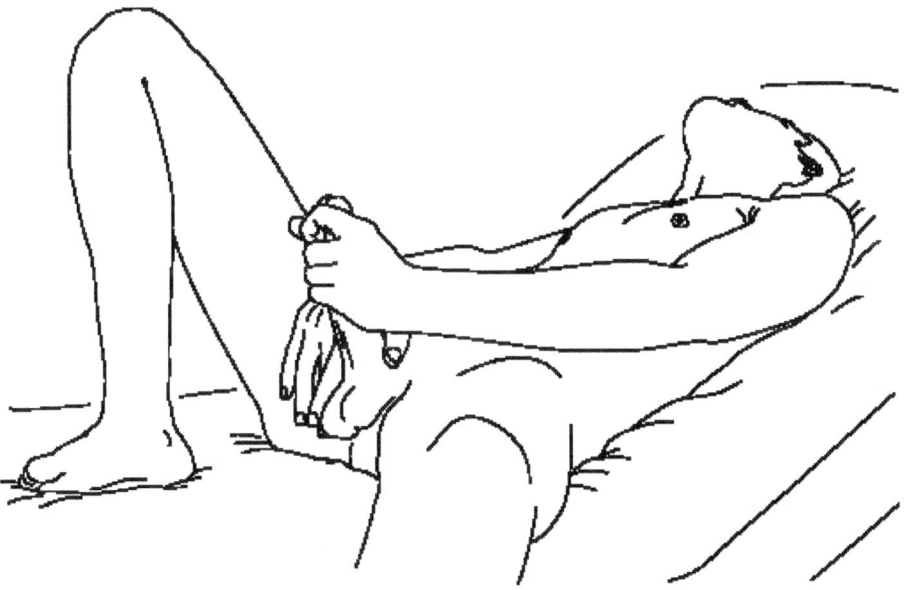

1. Begin in the standing position with your lubricated penis at the ready. You do not want to jelq with a fully erect penis, although most people will inevitably become aroused during the process.

Try to keep things at a level 1 or 2 hardness on the Erection Hardness Score – allow an erection to soften if it becomes too hard. Falling into masturbation will not be stretching the tissue out correctly as you'll be feeling for pleasure points and focusing more on the top of your penis.

2. Create a circle with the thumb and forefinger of your dominant hand. This may sometimes be called the 'okay' symbol. Loop this over your penis until it is resting at the base.

3. Pull up the length of the shaft away from your body while maintaining the loop – stop before you reach the glans of your penis. There should be some pressure applied here, but not so much that you are in any pain or discomfort, but not so light that no stretching could occur. This should take around 3 seconds for the first initial strokes.

4. Do not go backwards with the jelq and continue to begin at the base and pull away along the shaft. As you go on lengthen the time you take with each pull up to 10 seconds for one stroke. Repeat this process for 10 minutes maximum and try to aim for at least 10 minutes a day.

You can use alternate between hands to jelq for a smoother experience that goes for a fuller stretch. What you are trying to do is stretch the tissue out so it's fine to use different grips as long as they achieve that. However, the 'okay sign' is best as it applies consistent pressure and gives more a stretching motion.

Some practitioners recommend alternating up the angle you pull away too to give your penis a more throughout stretch – however, this is unnecessary unless you are trying to correct a curve. But, if you want to change the angle feel free to do so.

Should I get a Jelqing machine?

Various grips and wire vices have been created to help with Jelqing. Most of them are similar to eyebrow curlers for the penis, with a roller instead of a metal blade.

For the most part you do not need one of these machines as they do nothing that the average hand cannot, and you may be tempted to go harder than you need to with one.

The only exception might be if you struggle to create much pressure with your hands, or you have problems with carrying out repetitive motions with your hand. In which case, a Jelqing machine might make up for the shortfall of your hand.

Jelqing problems

If you are using skin-friendly lubricants, you warm-up fully, and you are not applying too much pressure it is very unlikely that you will encounter any problems at all when jelqing.

Some people have reported they created swelling at the end of their penis by doing this, or ended up with a misshapen, albeit longer, penis. This is very unlikely to happen, and would be the result of improper jelqing. Make sure that you cover the whole of the shaft with each pull and give yourself a break if you notice swelling.

Red spotting or rashes may occur for those who do not warm-up, do not lubricate, and apply too much pressure. If you are convinced you are not guilty of any of these things then you should considering trying a different method, using a different lubricant, or trying again after a 7-day hiatus.

Penis girth exercises

Jelqing may be the go-to exercise for many people, but it is not the only proven method of penis enlargement and it's primarily designed to increase length. For many men, they don't just want a longer penis – they want a penis with more girth.

With good reason, as several studies support the common theory that women find extra girth more pleasurable than length, as well as preferring the look of an imposing penis to a longer, skinnier one.

A study done at UCLA, where women handled 3D models of penises, women favored penis with a larger than average girth – especially when choosing a partner for a one night stand. When choosing a long term partner, surprisingly, girth and length were less important to women.

The theory is that a clitoris can be better stimulated with extra girth.

As with any exercise routines or techniques for working out one part of the body, which have many similarities, penis girth exercises are not radically different from penis lengthening exercises like jelqing. However, it is useful to master these techniques and use them in your workout schedule.

Flaccid Bend

The flaccid bend is a potentially trickier and more injury prone exercise, so you should be cautious when trying it out - have the motion nailed before you make it more intense or start doing lots of reps.

The basic idea of this exercise is, as the name implies, the bending of your penis to ensure that the tissue in the middle stretches outwards and not just lengthways.

You may want to use some lube for this exercise, but it's not entirely necessary. However, a warm-up is essential as you will want your penis to be as pliable as possible. This is a 'flaccid bend', so the penis should be as soft as you can manage and it should not be carried out with a penis is too hard to comfortable move and bend.

1. You can stand or sit for this exercise, and you begin by warming your penis in your hands and allowing for a very mild erect state, so there is more to work out.

2. Using one hand grab the glans of the penis like a doorknob, though not too hard, so that you have control over your penis. If you are sensitive here you may find some light lube helps a lot. Stretch out your penis to its full length without applying any painful pressure.

3. Place two fingers with the other hand at the base of your penis at the side facing away from you.

4. The idea is to bend your penis over the two fingers, and to hold it in place while bent. You are trying to stretch it flat rather than long, and the idea is to get some tension but to not hurt yourself in anyway. You are not bending your penis in half; so much as you are getting it to bulge. Hold in the bent position for 5 seconds each rep.

5. Continue to bend your penis as before, but alternate the angle left and right while moving your two fingers to different locations at the base of your penis.

You should try to do this exercise for 5 minutes each day and vary the length you bend your penis and the direction you do it to whatever is comfortable for you.

Belt Jelqing (or hand vice)

Belt jelqing is a variation on the standard jelq, but it is designed to focus primarily on girth by not just pushing upwards. Imagine squeezing a toothpaste tube from both ends – this is the kind of result you are trying to achieve here.

Lubricant will be vital for this exercise and you will need to practice more than with standard jelqing to ensure you are getting the right balance of movement, and not placing too much pressure on your penis.

1. Begin by standing and warm your penis up into a level 2 erection.

2. Turn the thumb and forefinger of both hands into the 'okay symbol', and then loop one around the base of your penis and loop the other around the head of your penis (just below the glans).

3. While firmly holding your penis with your hand at the base, bring down your other hand along the length of the shaft while squeezing.

4. Once the two hands have met squeeze your hand back up to the head of the penis. Hopefully, you will be able to feel the blood in your penis being pushed up and done the shaft and making extra girth in the tissue for when you do get an erection.

For this to work you will need a nearly erect penis or else you will struggle to complete a full rep. The movement should be firm and slow, taking around 5 seconds.

A more advanced version of this requires a penis clamp and we will explore that later in the guide. Belt jelqing, however, should be more than adequate for most people to increase the girth of their penis, and it can be used as an alternative jelqing technique.

Penis lengthening exercises

The Jelq is the classic penis length exercise, but that is also a general purpose exercise which will have some impact on girth. Here, we will look at exercises and techniques that can be used for targeted penis lengthening.

Jelqing should be your staple move, but if you really want to make gains on length, then try using some of these in your workout routine. Sometimes the effect on your penis will seem only subtly different, but that subtle difference may be enough to impact some erectile tissue that otherwise was left out.

You will find hundreds of variations of these techniques and exercises, but with the ones outlined in this guide you should have the knowledge to work-out the main areas of erectile tissue. Feel free to experiment, while staying safe, if you want to try different angles or variations of the exercises discussed here.

Two-handed five-finger Jelq

This technique goes by several names, but it is essentially just a jelq that uses two hands and is therefore more intense. It is important here that you lube up well as using two hands can create a lot more friction, and one of the biggest differences is that you do this technique while sat down.

This is a more concerted way of getting blood pumping along your shaft and you will want to be more patient with it.

1. Begin by sitting down, preferably with your legs crossed, and then work your penis into a level 2 erection.

2. Then place both hands around the penis shaft starting at the base, with one hand slightly higher than the other. You do not need to use the 'okay symbol' with this technique.

3. Move your hands slowly to the head of your penis (without touching the glans) and then move them away. This should take around 4 seconds.

4. Repeat this process from the base and take your hands away when you are done.

The pressure you apply should be firm and you are really trying to get the blood pushed up the length of your penis here, while taking up the whole body of the shaft. Be careful not to make this technique two hard as there is potential for injury if you do.

Twist and Pull

This is a technique that can help with both length and girth, but it's a fantastic technique to include in a routine because it works out a much wider range of erectile tissue. Lube is a must for this technique and you'll want to take it slowly as twisting can cause injury.

1. Get your penis close to a level 2 erection, longer but still pliable, and then twist it. To do this place a finger and thumb around the base and a finger and thumb just below the glans, then begin to slowly rotate your penis either clockwise or anti-clockwise until it has rotated around 90 degrees or far as you feel comfortable.

2. While in the same twisted position let go of the penis with the hand near the base and keep hold near the glans. Being to stretch the penis upwards until you have a firm, but comfortable, stretch achieved.

3. Hold your penis in the stretch for 5 seconds.

4. Let go of your penis and then repeat the process, this time twisting the penis in the opposite direction of the one you previously used.

When putting this technique into a routine keep it to a maximum of 5 minutes as it can be intense, and you don't want to end up with a sore penis.

Advanced Kegel Stretch

A kegel (or a PC muscle exercise) will flex the muscle running from your pubic bone to your tail bone, it is also able to exercise control over your penis and urethra.

Later we will discuss how to do kegel, and how they can be used in penis enlargement, but here we will be looking at how to use them in a specific penis lengthening technique. Carrying out a proper kegel takes some practice, but you should be able to achieve something similar by just flexing the muscle around your sphincter and genital areas.

What you are looking for here is the pulse of movement that you feel through your penis when you do this. You will use that to create a more powerful type of lengthening exercise. This is one that should not be carried out by beginners and it is best to practice kegels first.

You will not need a lot of lube for this to work, but you do need to warm up and have a comfortable work-out area to do them in. Despite being quite an involved technique, it is quite a simple one to follow.

1. You will need to be in a position where you can stretch you penis out straight – this will most likely be by standing, but you can even place your penis on a flat surface if you wish. You will need a level 2 erection for this technique.

2. Begin doing simple, rhythmic kegels that tense and relax along the base and shaft of your penis. Do this slowly so that you feel the tension in your penis for at least 2 seconds at a time.

3. Once you have the rhythm going begin gently stretching your penis out in different directions in time with the pulse of the kegel. If you like you can combine this with a quick jelq in the direction you choose.

Avoid doing this technique for too long as it can lead to penis fatigue – this will also count towards a daily kegel count if you are trying to increase your sexual performance.

Glans exercises

Many penis enlargement techniques and exercises focus primarily on the length of the shaft, and especially on working out the base or outer skin of the penis. In fact, the glans are specifically avoided in many exercises because they are sensitive and many feel they are already large enough.

The number of techniques that affect the size of your glans are limited, but here we will discuss the most powerful one and a variation on it. You might not feel like you need to do this, but you most likely want to keep a penis that looks in proportion so consider working it into your routine every few days at least.

Pressure Bulb Squeeze

This is a simple exercise that can cause injury if it is done vigorously – so practice caution and go only so long as you are comfortable. The idea is to trap blood in a full erection and force it to increase the size of the head of the penis.

Lubricant is not required for this exercise and due to the hardness of the erection required in can be a good way to finish an exercise routine.

1. Get your penis to a level 4 erection and take a standing or loose sitting position.

2. Make the 'okay symbol' with your dominant hand and loop it around the base of your penis. Make sure you have a firm grip of your penis.

3. Begin squeezing your penis so that you can feel the blood trapped. Consider doing a kegel before tightening your grip.

4. Hold for 5 to 7 seconds, release and then repeat for up to 3 minutes.

Using the squeeze you shouldn't struggle too much with maintaining a harder erection. If you do then pause to work it back up, but avoid focusing too much on the pleasure and forgetting what you are here to do.

Advanced Bulb Squeeze

The advanced bulb squeeze is very similar to the previous technique; it simply uses your other hand to squeeze even tighter. You should move on to this stage once you are more familiar with the level of pressure your can happily apply and how to better control the blood flow in your penis.

1. Get your penis to a level 4 erection and take a standing or loose sitting position.

2. Make the 'okay symbol' with your dominant hand and loop it around the base of your penis. Make sure you have a firm grip of your penis.

3. Take your other hand and loop it just below the head of your penis and squeeze just as tight.

4. Begin squeezing your penis so that you can feel the blood trapped. Begin by squeezing with the hand at the base and then begin squeezing with the other when blood has risen higher to keep it nearer the glans.

5. Hold for 5 to 7 seconds, release and then repeat for up to 3 minutes.

Considering only doing the advanced technique every so often and keep the amount of time shorter to avoid penis fatigue.

Penis straightening exercises

On its own having a straighter penis will not increase length, but a curved penis can make a penis look shorter, and some people feel uncomfortable with what they perceive as an abnormal looking penis.

When talking about penis curvature, it usually means too far to the left or right – slight variation are perfectly normal and should not be a concern, but too much of a bend might need correction. If you are experiencing painful curvature you should consult a doctor.

Many of the other techniques in this guide will help with straightening, but the two techniques listed here will specifically looking to helping you get a straighter penis.

These will need to be done daily for a full effect and you should not expect dramatic changes as stretching and lifting weights may not be enough to change the underlying cause of a curved penis. Expect changes to be shorter term, as you simply can't stretch your penis permanently in any one direction (in the way you can stretch it so that it's longer).

Curve-correction Pull

This technique is a lot like a basic jelq, the only difference is that you are intentionally correcting for curvature in the penis. For this to work better you will need a harder penis and be slightly firmer than you would with a jelq.

Rather than trying to stretch tissue for a longer penis, you are trying to get it to stand straight and this can be done with a stretch also, but it's more like setting a mold.

1. Begin in a standing position and get a level 3 erection.

2. Put your thumb and forefinger in an 'okay symbol' and loop around the base of your penis.

3. Firmly pull your hands up the shaft of your penis and pull in the opposite direction of the curve. Be firm while doing this so there is definite movement. It should take you 3 to 4 seconds to make this move.

4. Hold your penis in this position with your hand now below the glans. Try to trace the blood along the shaft so you can hold it there in place. Don't worry about getting your penis to be in your desired straight position; you can curve further the other way to counter-balance the current curvature.

If you are interested in a straighter penis then you might consider using this technique instead of the standard jelq, just make sure to equally squeeze the shaft and then trap blood in the top of your penis while you hold the correction curve.

Pelvic exercises

Pelvic exercises are not essential for an enlarged penis – however they can help greatly with sexual performance and will increase your overall fitness, as well as your control over your penis.

Getting a larger penis is not always just about stretching out the tissue so there is more penis to get hard – it's also about ensuring you can get the fullest erection possible, and you have the ability to improve sexual performance.

By increasing the strength of your pelvis you'll be able to manually give yourself stiffer erections and maintain it at its full strength for longer. The pelvic exercises are probably the most energy consuming of the exercises in this guide, so make sure to warm up and to improve your overall fitness while you work on them.

Towel Deadlift

The concept behind this exercise is very simple and when done regularly it can dramatically increase the strength of your pelvis. The main caveat is that you can over-strain yourself with this and cause permanent injury.

It works by having you lift a towel with your erect penis for several reps. How heavy the towel is will be left up to you, and you may want to opt for a heavier towel as your PC muscles get stronger. A tea towel is probably too light, but a full beach towel may cause real fatigue or pain. By doing this exercise your pubococcygeus muscles will get a work-out and give you a stiffer erection.

No lube is required for this and you should start with as few as 20 reps and work your way up as you get stronger and more confident.

1. You will need to be in a position where you can easily lift a towel with your penis. This may be over a table, or standing for a smaller towel.

2. Get your penis to a level 4 erection and then place the towel over the shaft of the penis. The towel must rest on the penis so that it is able to lift it up.

3. As you breathe in, use your pelvic muscles to tense your penis and lift the towel. Once raised as high as possible hold for 3 seconds and then allow your penis to lower the towel.

4. Repeat this process for 50 to 100 reps.

If you are doing kegel exercises regularly, you may not need the towel deadlift in your arsenal, but it can be a fun way to alter up your routine and it can give you that extra work out.

Trampoline Exercises

This is not a specific technique so much as an action you can do to increase blood flow and workout your pelvis in a fun way.

As the name implies the idea is to get a workout on a trampoline. This does not have to be a large outdoor trampoline, as there smaller exercise ones available for the home, and many gyms have trampolines available for use as well as trampoline exercise classes.

If you wish, you can also do some basic bouncing exercises, such as jumping jacks, which will also help your pelvic muscles. Alternatively, an old spring mattress can be used in place of a trampoline – if you have one in the basement or garage, this might be a chance to get some use out of it.

There are many trampoline exercises which are great for both muscle building and cardio, but here we are interested in ones that exercises the pelvis – and this means bouncing.

*You can start with some simple bounces and **jumping jacks** to warm-up, then try a **standing bounce** where you go from sitting to standing as fast as possible; and, finally, try **plyo jumps** where you stand on one foot then switch to the other at the other side of the trampoline.*

If you do not have the desired privacy for full penis workouts every day then this trampoline can be a fantastic way to strengthen your pelvis and penis discreetly. Try to get in up to 30 minutes of cardio each day, and use the trampoline for a substantial part of that.

Kegels and PC Muscle Exercises

The concept of a kegel, the working out of your pelvis muscles, has become very popular in the last ten years. They've been adopted by the medical community as a fantastic way of increasing overall fitness, of reducing incontinence, improving sexual performance, and combating erectile dysfunction.

You may have seen PC muscle exercises being touted as well, but they are largely identical to kegels in execution. For some, despite the huge benefits to your penis and sex life, kegels are seen as feminine. Physiologically, however, men and women are similar enough that kegels benefit both.

Here we will refer to them as 'kegels', simply because it's a much easier way to talk about this specific exercise technique.

How do kegels work?

Of all the penis enhancement techniques, kegels are probably the best researched and there is a lot of evidence that it helps with erectile dysfunction and can help you control premature ejaculation.

They work by getting you to contract and then relax the muscles in your pelvis – known as the pelvic floor, or the pubococcygeus – a muscle going from your pubic bone to your coccyx. Both men and men have this muscle and can exercise them.

Your pelvis (or pelvic diaphragm) all works to relax and contract as part of the one muscle, so when you do this exercise you are strengthening your entire pelvic area. When you begin doing them you will feel the strain in your penis and you can even begin to practice by just stopping and starting the flow of urine when you go to pee.

By doing this you have already identified the mechanism and the muscle you will need to work out.

Having better control over this part of your body means you can flex your penis, you can encourage extra blood to be sent to it, you can hold on to a stiffened penis for longer, and stop ejaculate leaving the urethra easier.

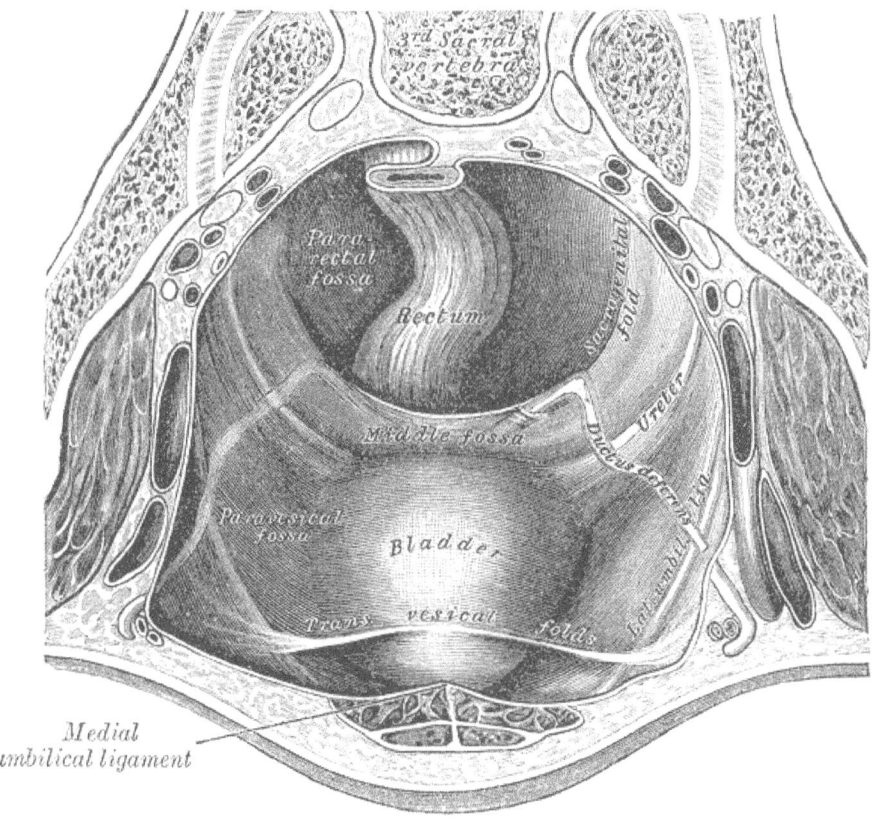

How to do a Kegel

To begin have a go at flexing or contracting the muscle mentioned in the last section – doing so while urinating is the easiest demonstration. Keep your leg and upper body muscles relaxed and focus on controlling your pelvic area.

Once you've learned how to reliably stop and start urination you have the basic kegel exercise down. To take this to a workout regime, do the kegel and when you're contracting the muscle keep it held like that for two to three seconds and then relax. Repeat this five to ten times a day to begin with.

The beauty of the kegel is that you can do them almost anywhere – even when sat at work or watching television. Put a timer or reminder on each day so that you can be sure to get them done. A commute to work is a perfect time to get your ten a day in.

Slowly you want to start adding longer and more kegels into your workout sessions. Try to make each Kegel last 10 seconds and double the amount of reps – every two weeks you should look to increase the length and number of kegels until you are doing 50 reps up to 3 times a day.

You can also try to do a more advanced kegel by doing a steady tremble kegel; start off with a small mild flex, then keep increasing the intensity and hold it for as long as 30 singles. Alternatively, go up the scales of intensity, start with a light kegel and keep going until you are at a full clench.

One rep with the more advanced kegels should count for three reps of a normal kegel. Which you choose to do should not matter enormously, as what's important is the regular exercise and build up of exercise.

When will I see results with kegels?

After the first month you should begin to feel a noticeable difference with your control over your PC muscles, and in 3 months you should feel much more control.

Like any exercise for muscle strength, if you stop then you will lose that strength – however, you might not need to be so intense after the first 6 months. There is a limit to how strong your PC muscles can get, or how strong you would even need them to be, so there is no need to do more than 50 reps a day for the vast majority of people.

Avoid doing too many kegels, especially early on. You will feel the strain if you push yourself too far, and injury is possible if go too hard or too strong (though injury will almost certainly never happen during normal kegels).

If you have a history of problems with your pelvis (or have recently had a hernia) then consult a doctor before adopting a full workout regime.

If you want a fuller penis thanks to your kegels then it's a good idea to get some practice in when you are erect, and also during masturbation or sexual intercourse.

First, begin by trying out a basic kegel while you have an erection. This is fairly simple and you should notice a bit more resistance, while also getting a fuller erection.

The next step is to try this during masturbation. This can be particularly fun if you try it with the technique known as 'edging'. Bring yourself close to ejaculation (or orgasm), and then stop and perform a kegel and hold it for a while. Repeat for several erections and when you do allow yourself to orgasm it should feel more intense. This should prime you for longer sex and teach you how to use your PC muscles in action.

You can do this during sex as well, but let your partner know what you are trying out. You might even want to encourage them to practice kegels at the same time.

Some men may experience a condition informally known as, 'blue balls' if they are aroused for a long time and continue to deny orgasm while semen has to run back into the testes. The usual cure is to achieve orgasm or wait out the pain.

Do I need a kegel device?

A general rule of thumb with any device related to penis enlargement is that it should be clear that the device does something you aren't already able to do.

Most kegel devices either don't help to exercise the pelvic floor, or don't enhance what you can already do. Save your money for a stretching device that will truly enhance what you can accomplish with penis enlargement.

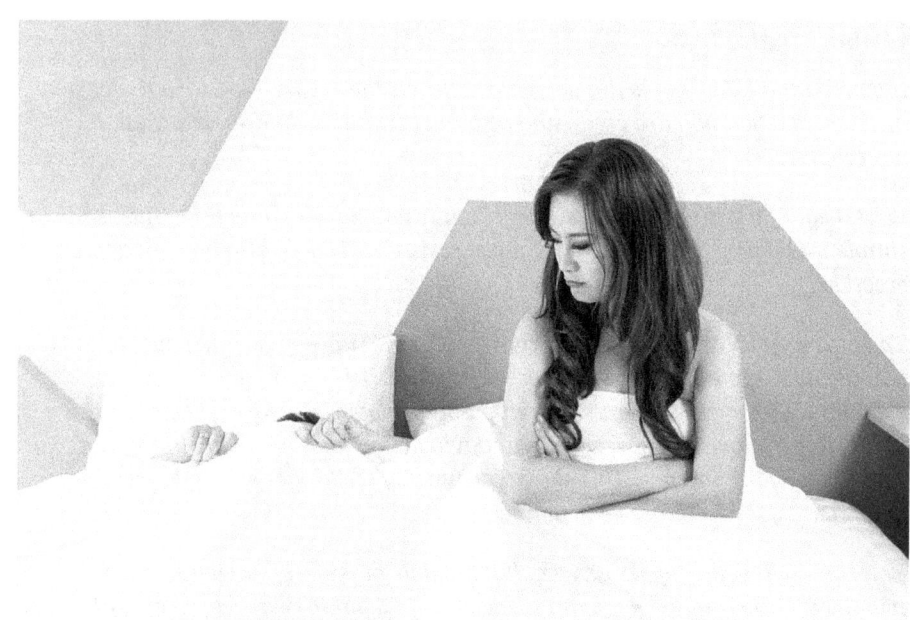

Health Supplements – Penis Pills, Herbs and Lotions

Out of all the penis enlargement products on the market which have questionable effects on the body – penis health supplements are the trickiest to get the truth on.

When you're out shopping for the many varieties of 'blue pills' or 'penis growing lotions,' it's not often clear how they will work, or even how they could work. However, pills do exist which can fight erectile dysfunction and increase penis length, as well as pills that can alter hormones in the body. Here we're going to tell you what to look out for.

What can you expect from penis supplements?

To begin with we should look at what you shouldn't expect from penis supplements; primarily this is not expecting a pill or lotion to get your penis to grow by itself.

Not only can no medicine do this exactly, but you would most likely want to avoid this - accelerated growths in the body could lead to serious health problems or cancer.

The penis has neither hard muscle nor bone in it, so to get it to grow you would need some kind of medicine that could expand tissue in the body, and would be able to specifically target erectile tissue. That simply cannot be done and any claims that it can without evidence should be ignored.

If we had pills that could make precision growths in the body, then you would see pills available for just about every body part. The body isn't magical though, and it can only work with the functions it already has.

What can expect from penis supplements, however, is to greatly enhance the penis growing techniques you are going to otherwise be doing, and to also increase erection size and sexual performance.

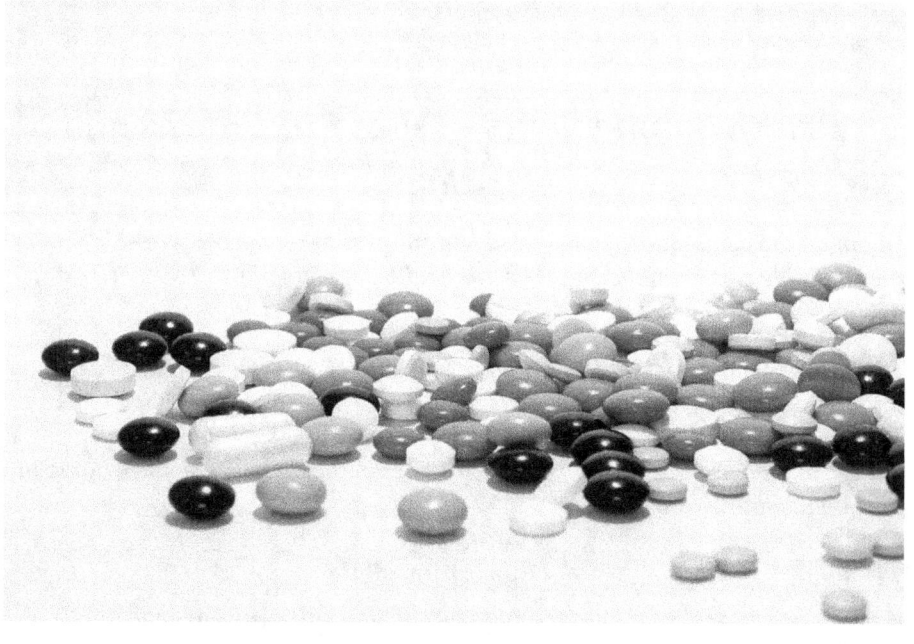

The three types of penis supplements

With this in mind there are two broad types of penis supplements you might consider.

Hormones

The first is to take specific hormones that help with speeding up body regeneration and encourage growth of male sex qualities. The main contender would be human growth hormones, such as somatotropin, which are what the body uses to regenerate cells, to regulate metabolism, and allows humans to grow during childhood.

Getting hold of HGH without a legitimate medical need is very difficult and not really advised. Heightened levels of HGH can lead to tumors and thicken bones in the jaw and hands causing serious health problems. In addition, they won't make your penis grow larger on their own; however, they will help with weight loss, muscle growth, and can speed up the growth of tissue. But with penis enlargement you are often looking to stretch tissue, rather than grow it.

You can find 'HGH releasers', on the market which do not contain growth hormones, but claim to help produce them quicker in the body. Evidence about their efficacy is scant – yet many claim they work well and they could certainly help with weight loss and fitness routines.

Testosterone is the other big name that goes around, and simply put it will not make your penis larger and it is unlikely to be of much benefit to you. Higher testosterone levels correspond to things such as muscle and hair growth – and can start puberty in some people.

However, there are limits to how much testosterone your body needs and it will naturally balance it out by not producing its own if it perceives it already has enough. This is why infamously it can shrink testicles – once your body has too much artificially it actually stops producing the hormone altogether.

Muscle relaxants

These are the health supplements that will do the best job of help your penis enlargement routine. They work by relaxing muscles and arteries around the pelvis and allowing more blood to flow into your penis.

The main medicine used for this is Sildenfail, or, as it's branded in most countries, 'Viagra'. Contrary to popular belief, this drug does not make you hornier or increase your libido; it simply allows blood to get into the penis more easily once you begin the process of getting an erection.

Many of the causes of erectile dysfunction, particularly nerves and high blood pressure, can be alleviated with this medicine. Since your aim is to trap blood in your penis and use it to change and stretch the tissue inside these drugs are also of value during exercise routines and in getting a harder erection.

Viagra is quite a potent drug, and just for use in penis enlargement is unnecessary and also not fantastic to have too often. In addition it will also require a prescription – as will similar drugs like Cialis or tadalafil.

Luckily, there are several alternatives and even natural compounds that have been proven to create a similar effect in the body. The most well known of these alternatives, are Horny Goat Weed, Macca, Cordycepys, and Red Ginseng.

Mood and health enhancers

Finally these are the truly supplementary supplements. Several drugs and medicines can increase your ability to lose, feel active, gain muscle, and even improve your mood and consequently your libido.

The list of these drugs is enormous and not many are specifically useful for penis enlargement, but they are fantastic for giving your routine a boost. As is a good diet, which is full of nutrients, slow-burning energy, and avoids low or high blood-pressure, and discourages gall stones. Meaning, you should avoid too much salt or saturated fat in your diet. Nuts and small amounts of alcohol have been shown to help prevent gall stones.

What to avoid

The simple rule is to avoid anything without active ingredients proven to do any of the above mentioned functions. Check the ingredients on supplements and ensure the main ingredients have some proven efficacy.

Price should not be a huge factor here, as the basic chemical should do the same thing no matter the label, but you may be able to be more cost-effective with pills that do more than one thing and give you several nutrients.

Lotions and creams tend to not be fantastic ways of helping penis growth, even if they have the right ingredients in them. Administering these things as creams is typically troublesome when you are trying to treat an issue that is below the skin.

Moisturizers and skin-healing creams may be of some use to you, however they will just improve the appearance or softness of your penis – not its length or girth.

Best over the counter supplements to use

Check with a trusted supplier for drugs that meet your needs and consult a doctor before trying too much of any particular supplement – especially if you have health concerns.

This guide recommends the _Mr. Thick_ and advanced Horny _Goat Weed pills_ created by USA supplements. They are reasonably priced and come in a large bottle that will keep you well stocked during your regime.

Both contain ingredients like _Maca and Horny Goat Weed_ which will give you the main impact of extra blood in your penis, and they also contain energy boosting extras like Ginseng that will help with your work-out.

Mr. Thick even has L-Arginine in it which can encourage testosterone production. While it's not a brilliant idea to regularly take pure testosterone on its own, as you get older your testosterone productions levels will begin to drop, and by topping this up you can gain muscle quicker and should hasten penis enlargement.

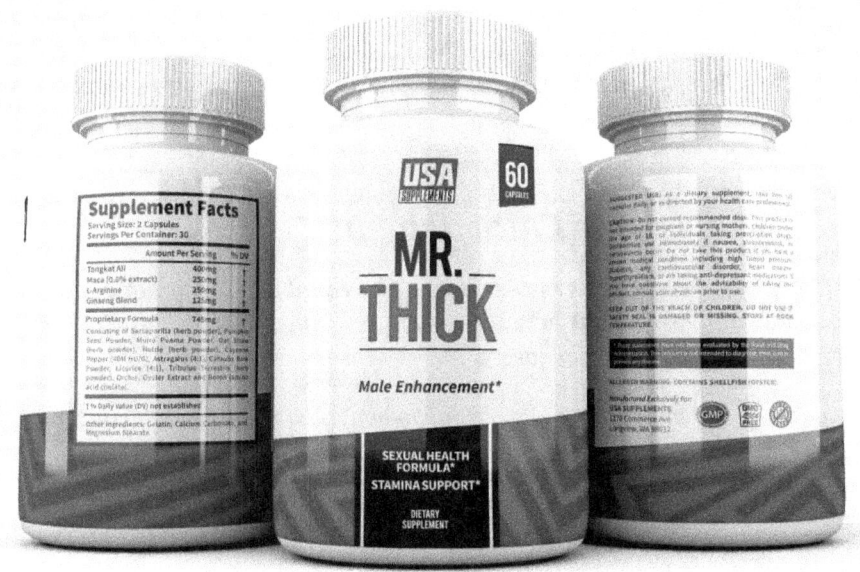

If you are using health boosters and muscle relaxants then you will want to use them in conjunction with your work-out routine. Follow the recommended dosage and try to make sure you use them before you work-out to get the full impact.

The main use is in having extra blood in your penis so that you can squeeze and pull with more efficiency. A supplement like Mr. Thick is made to be taken daily, so it should work ideally with your routine.

Taking the supplements too late in the day or after you've worked-out can make them less effective. In addition, you should be careful about using the supplements and doing exercises such as kegels in public as that can lead to some embarrassing situations.

When you want to show off your hard work – make sure to take the supplements first, at least an hour or two before sexual activity. It should provide you with more energy and a harder erection.

Penis Enlargement Devices

The world of penis enlargement devices can be equal parts weird and wonderful, and this guide is here to talk you through what works, what doesn't, and what should be made illegal.

If you are very serious about penis enlargement on a permanent basis then one or two of the devices here are a must as part of your regime. Not only do they really work, but they are just about the only way to make serious gains in a reasonable time without dangerous surgery.

With the right guidance you can increase erection size, stretch your penis longer than you can by hand, and also improve the appearance of your penis.

How can a penis enlargement device help me?

For the most part penis enlargement devices work by boosting the principles discussed in the various exercises. They either try to stretch the penis tissue or, in some instances, they will stretch the length of the skin on your penis. Some work essentially like a cock ring, and help to keep extra blood in the penis whilst you do exercises.

The most famous enlargement device is no doubt the penis pumper, and this works too, to increase the blood in the penis and can be a useful penis enlargement device.

Where some devices fail is in not actually stretching the penis tissue, or in doing nothing your hand can't, or just bizarrely massaging your penis for no true possibility of growth or change.

The types of penis enlargement devices

There are a few broad groups of penis enlargement devices to look out for and we'll run down the main categories here.

Extenders and Traction devices

Penis extenders are probably the most popular type of penis enlargement device – and with good reason. It's a safe and easy option, while also having some considerable scientific backing behind it.

They way it works, is by having you place your penis in a kind of stretcher that is made of two extendable rods. The head is fixed in place and then you can stretch it out for an extended period of it.

Weights and Hanging

Hanging was the original penis enlargement method of choice and its use has a history dating back hundreds of years in some cultures.

The apparatus is very simple – you put a sheath of some kind around your penis and then hang weights off it. It's a little more complex than just stretching, but it has proven results.

The downside, as you might imagine, is that anchoring down your penis with weights can be a dangerous and uncomfortable if not done correctly.

Clamps

This device work much like a cock ring by trapping more blood in the penis, so that it can become fuller and in theory stretch and grow bigger. These are usually used in conjunction with exercises, rather than doing too much on their own.

There's less evidence for their efficacy versus just using your hand, however they are often cheap and do serve a purpose that isn't negligible.

Pressure Pumps and Vacuums

These devices use the pressure created either from water or air to trap extra blood in the penis. On one level they function similar to a clamp, however they also work to enlarge the body.

You can see for yourself that pressure can be used to enlarge parts of the body, and certainly these devices work to help gain an erection, and a fuller erection; the idea is that your fuller erection will then stretch out your penis long term.

Devices to avoid

It would be too simplistic to say avoid any device that doesn't into one off the categories above, but that might be a rule of thumb you want to consider.

A better rule to follow is to ask: "is there any logical way this could make my penis larger?" If the answer is a resounding "no", then it's best to avoid the product altogether.

There are many excellent customer advice comparisons sites and reviews aggregates that will tell you what to avoid. However, there are also many professional looking websites that will tell you outright lies about research they've done or what a product can do.

You should expect all devices to exaggerate a little in the kind of growth the average person could expect from them (those tests are always based on someone using the device perfectly and punctually). But if the claims go too far and you can't find anything to back them up (from a more neutral source), then assume it won't make your penis 12 inches longer. Some claims are too good to be true.

There are no secret answers to penis enlargement and the popular solutions are popular for a reason.

Crystals and magnets are probably the biggest offenders of strange penis extending devices. Magnet therapy has no evidence behind it, and anyone that tells you wearing a bikini-bottom full of magnets will make your penis larger has lost their mind.

Electric therapy is another device that has no chance of making your penis larger. You can zap your balls all day long if you want, but the best you can hope for is a more intense orgasm or a lower sperm count.

You will need to also look out for devices that are overcomplicated or impractical. You can find all kinds of rings and shiny things to places around your penis, but if they don't do anything that a basic clamp or extender wouldn't – then you don't need one.

There are some devices that might potentially work, but should, nevertheless, be avoided. These are devices that strap your penis to your knee, or help you bend it half-war around your hips. There is no justification to putting yourself in this kind of discomfort.

The worst crime many of these devices commit is simply being too silly, but some of them could genuinely bring you harm. In the wild west of the internet, there is no real regulation about what inventions can be sold. Attaching electrical nodes down the length of your penis with some torture device you've bought with Chinese-only instructions is a bad idea.

Penis Extender

The first device we're going to look at is arguably the most prevalent in the penis enlargement community. Sometimes the method is referred to as 'penis traction', but they all do largely the same thing.

Nearly all of the devices look the same, and have a reassuring clinical look about them. When you first look at them you might think they would be painful, as you are stretching your penis out with a metal rod. However, the tension they create is surprisingly gentle and can be easily folded into your daily life.

Many of the devices are well engineered and well-built pieces of equipment, so make sure to do the spade work before you buy. It's easy to end up with a cheap knock-off that will break very quickly, but a better model will often only cost you a little extra.

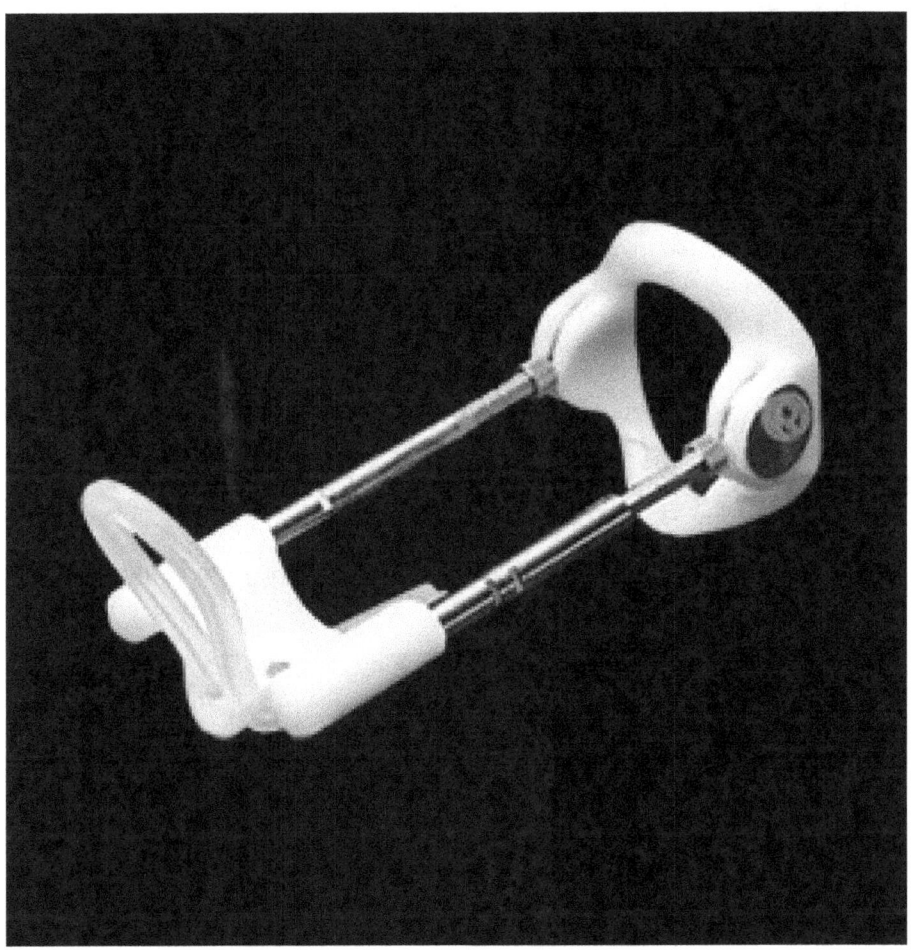

How they work

An extender has two plastic ends connected by two telescopic rods. One end is an arch or loop that can be slotted comfortably around the base of the penis, and the other is built more like a cradle where the head of the penis can be rested.

The head is strapped into the cradle and then the rods are extended so your penis is being stretched. You then wear the extender for your chosen stretching period and some models will let you happily wear it with your trousers on over the top (though there is a good chance a bulge will be on display).

This is done while the penis is flaccid and can be done for up to an hour a day. The only constraint is that you can't do too much exercise while wearing it.

Most models will allow you to keep extending the rod to accommodate a lengthened penis, and will easily retract for much short penises. Some also claim to be able to help straighten your penis (though there's less evidence that it will accomplish this as well as lengthening).

This is the basic mechanism of all extenders and the difference between devices is nearly entirely about how it cradles the head of your penis. Some use a very simple strap over a wide cradle. Others use tubing or quite an intense grip. The more sophisticated devices have a cap that is pumped on to the glans of the penis and this is held by the device without a true cradle at all.

Many users will want to use some kind of grip or gauze to prevent any damage or marks on the penis from extended use.

With this method the penis tissue is stretched and the same kind of tearing that occurs with muscle building should occur, so that your penis actually re-grows in this new lengthened state.

Step-by-step safe usage

You won't need lube to use the penis extender and you want a flaccid penis to level 1 erection. A full erection won't be possible when the device is on and the restraints should stop one from happening.

Warm-up exercises are a good idea when you are getting started with the extender so you can be your full length and pliable. Avoid using an extender if you have any skin conditions on your penis (such as jock itch) as this might exacerbate some symptoms.

Some extenders will require you to set-up the device yourself – this is just a simple matter of screwing in the rods in most instances. When you start using it, begin with the cradle not extended.

1. Depending on the type of extender you have you may or may not want to put some kind of padding around the glans – or area of the penis that will be in the cradle of the device. Some extender kits provide a protective pad for you to use.

2. Prepare the device for placing your penis on it. This might mean getting the strap ready in place with one hand.

3. Place the head of your penis in the cradle – you may be more comfortable having the cradle touching the area just below the glans. You won't lose out on significant growth by doing it this way.

4. Tighten the strap until you feel a tension in your penis. It should not be painful or oppressive, but you should definitely feel secure and as though your penis will be stretched and not just laying in this contraption.

5. When you are securely fitted in then you can begin to adjust the rods until your penis is being stretched. You do not need a painful stretch at all and you will not be speeding up the stretching process by doing so. For growth you simply need a stretch, and so you should stick to a comfortable one.

Maintain this stretch for up to an hour and as you start to see growth you will naturally be readjusting the length of the stretch. Remember to be hygienic here and to store the device in a place that it will not get too damp.

How long you wish to use the device will be up to you. As with muscles, if you stop using it for a long period of time you might see a reversal in your gains, but not too dramatic of a reduction.

Some users will use the extender for as many as 6 hours a day, while making sure to have 30 minute breaks between hour long sessions. That is quite an intense workout and depending on your lifestyle may be too much. An hour or two a day should be fine.

Expect to start seeing real results after around two months and expect your penis to become accustomed to regular stretching after around six months.

If things are getting painful stop using the device or begin stretching it less. If you find you are getting blisters, rashes, or other painful results then consider using the device less or trying out a new type of cradle.

Which device to buy

Some of the penis extension devices can get very expensive and some will come with superfluous attachments that you don't necessarily need to see real improvement.

There is a lot of marketing speak going around with the various devices and talk about multi-way 'comfort systems'. The truth is that as long as you have a protective pad then you shouldn't have an issue.

This guide recommends going for a tubular strap over a rubber strap (as they are slightly more comfortable), but both options are fine and it will come down to your personal preference).

If you are looking for a rubber strap model then try the MaleEdge or Size Genetics. If you are looking for a tube strap then try the JES extender or the Quick Extender Pro.

The PeniMaster Pro does things a little differently by giving you a vacuum cap for the head of your penis and is much better if you want to be mobile and free to move around while you are using your penis extender. The Phallosan forte has a similar sheath for your penis if you do not want to use a traditional cradle.

Many users prefer a vacuum seal as they feel it is more comfortable – especially when wearing the device for a long period of time. However, expect to pay more for the vacuum option. If you plan to use the device every day it may be a worthwhile investment.

Penis Pal is one of the cheaper extenders on the market and comes with a simple but efficient tubular strap. You should see the same results with a device like this – you just may need to buy your own protective pads and will have less flexibility for options.

How to use them in your enlargement regime

A penis extender can work to replace the need for some exercises. They will provide enough stretching on their own that doing long drawn out stretches yourself is not necessary because you can just use the extender.

If you are interested in just extra length and you are happy to use one for two hours a day, then it can do most of the leg work. However, the extender does work mostly on a flaccid penis and you will want to compliment it with exercises that increase blood flow and help to lengthen an erection.

Realistically you can't spend several hours a day working out just your penis, and you won't be able to work out while using the extender. What you will need to do is use supplement for the extra blood flow and then do some powerful exercises for at least 30 minutes a day.

The jelqin should be fine for this and if you do kegels you can try for a fuller erection when you need it. Jelqins can also be useful to let you put extra blood back into your penis after you have been using the extender for a while.

Extenders to avoid

The majority of penis extenders available on the market are safe to use, and shouldn't cause you any problems. However, a few of the cheaper and stranger designs should be avoided.

You need an extender that uses metal rods and not one that working with a plastic sliding mechanism, like some kind of telescope for your penis. These will give you less control over the amount of stretch you have and will require you to more or less stay in the same position while you use them.

More importantly, you need to look out for extenders that use cheap or harsh chords to keep your penis within the extender cradle. These could cause serious welts or damage to your penis if you are not careful.

Penis Hanging

Penis hangers are the other main method of penis extension and many prefer them to the extenders as they typically do not require you to use them for as long to see results.

The process is almost as simple as the name implies. You attach a harness near the head of your penis and then hang weights off it. Many people then start doing exercises to increase the impact of the weights.

The hanging both stretches the penis, and does exercises that can help lengthen the tissue of the penis.

The reason you need a device for this, is that simply hanging weights off your penis with a piece of string would be likely to cause you problems. It can be done safely and effectively, but only with the right training and equipment.

How it works

The growing mechanism being triggered with the hanger is very similar to the one with the extender (which is why extenders are often the device of choice for many).

By pulling your penis down you create a strain and this creates tiny tears that will heal back up, but longer along the lines of the tears. But, don't worry, the tears will heal back to normal skin (and won't be noticeable as they tear), resulting in a permanently longer penis.

Technically, this is just how stretching skin and body tissue works – it's the same with your nose or earlobes. However, your penis is able to grow and stretch thanks to the soft muscle in it.

To safely penis hang you'll need some kind of sheath for your penis that will allow you to hold a weight, while also using the heft of your penis to lift it. All penis hanging works with the same principle, but different devices allow weights to be hung in different ways, and they can allow you to use more weights.

One of the advantages of penis hanging is that you can increase the amount of weights and keep stretching your penis longer. There is a much higher limit to the amount of length you can add. Hanging does primarily increase length, but it can also help straighten your penis.

The big risk, of course, is that if you hang too much weight you will cause considerable damage to your penis. In addition if you too much, too quickly – then you can stretch your penis too fast and it will not have the appearance you desire.

Most devices recommend you do a 2 to 3 months of training before using penis hanging, and you begin with 2 to 5 pound weights – adding 1 to 2 pounds a week, till the point you are uncomfortable or you've achieved your lengthening goals. Pros can get up to 25 pounds. You'll do this for 20 to 30 minutes up to three times a week, with one day of rest between. Here, you can see part of the appeal of hanging – since it's much quicker than extending.

For the first few weeks you'll notice mostly skin stretching around the penis, but after the first 2 or 3 weeks there should be an increase of the penis tissue.

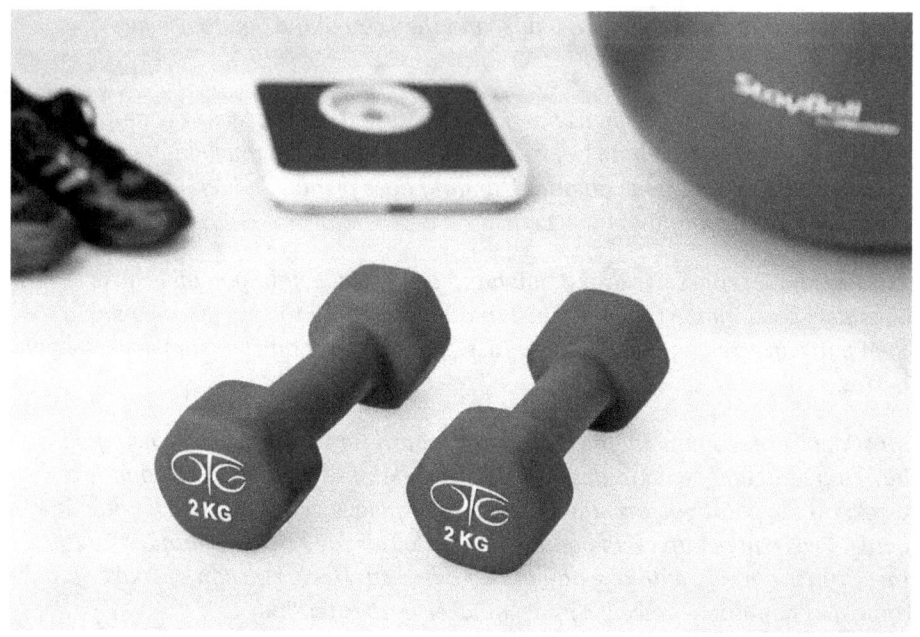

Step-by-step safe usage

How you apply the weights will depend on the device you buy, but here we'll look at a basic vacuum hanger with a rubber sleeve. Most devices do now use a vacuum seal, but some use a simple noose.

To begin you'll want to warm-up considerably so that you are nice and loose; however, using lubricant is not necessary here. Your penis should be flaccid while you do this and will not work if you begin to get erect while placing the device on.

No matter how much experience you get or how much weight you feel comfortable in hanging, always start slowly and add the weight on a few pounds at a time. Some users like to tape (using micropore tape) or bandage up their glans to reduce the risk of swelling or blistering.

1. Get in a comfortable standing position and take the device with both hands. Roll bag the rubber sheath back until there is only the dome at the end of the device, then place the head of your penis in the dome.

2. At this point you can start pumping air into the dome with the vacuum to start creating pressure. You can then unfurl the rubber sheath down the length of your penis towards the base. The vacuum is being used to make suction so you can keep the device on easily – it should be comfortably around 5 gs (the pressure meter should show you where it's at).

3. Attach the weight to the hook or carabineer, use your hands or the floor so the weight is taken on gently, and only add what you are comfortable hanging.

4. You can simply stand with the strain for a 20 minute rep. You are trying to reach a level of fatigue with your penis, and you might find doing some mild kegels helps. If you get fatigued before the 20 minutes is up you may stop early.

 You can increase the number of reps you do a day, but you must always take at least a 10 minute break between reps. Jelqs will help here to get blood back into your penis.

To stay safe stop if there is any pain. You should not be experiencing pain during this exercise (though fatigue is not pain), and any sharp pain is an indication you need to stop immediately or lower the amount of weights being used.

Which device to buy

There is more variety with hangers than extenders, and your personal preference is more important here. You have to choose a type of device depending on how you want it to attach to your penis, and the kind of weights you want to use.

Traditional hanger

There are broadly two types of hangers available. There is the traditional hanger, often known as bib hangers, and they work by creating a loop to be placed just below the glans of the penis with a hook hanging below.

The only thing keeping them in place is the grip created around the penis and you will almost certainly need padding for them to be comfortable. The most popular devices use what is essentially a vice that is clamped around your penis with some nuts and bolts. Despite looking a bit daunting, these hangers nearly *always come with padding and are relatively comfortable to have one once you get the adjustments right for you.*

BibHanger is the most famous and arguably the most popular brand of traditional hanger or you may want to try the simpler and cheaper MaleHanger (though it is also lacking in sophistication).

Other devices like the Zen Hanger work more like a noose for your penis, and would theoretically grip around below the glands with a soft piece of cloth or padding underneath. On first inspection these devices might seem like they would be more comfortable, but here most of the weight would be taken by the glans and there is huge room for injury or accidents.

Vacuum hanger

The main alternative to the tradition grip is the vacuum hanger. These work by placing the head of your penis in a plastic or silicone dome that can have a pump attached to it. You can then increase the pressure so the hanger stays comfortably on your penis.

This attachment will then have some kind of sheath or sleeve that will roll up the rest of your penis shaft. Most people will find the vacuum hanger is the most comfortable; however, it can only take so much weight before it falls off. If you are planning on putting over 25 pounds on your penis then a traditional hook is the better option.

LG Hanger is the most popular brand around and it comes with a well-built rubber sheath and lots of online support for its use.

Penis weight

The third option is not truly a hanger, but you can buy individual penis weights that come with a loop attached and can carry a few pounds of weight. These are generally not very practical (as they can come off easily), and they will not allow you to do a full hanging exercise.

However, if you want a mild weight on your penis then this might a tangible option. Some of the more bizarre weights have several loops along the penis shaft where you can attach weights. This is unlikely to do anything for you penis so avoid them.

When it comes to weights for the other hangers you will have a choice of disk weights, fishing weights, and even a type of dumbbell. Your choice will depend on the hanger you choose and how you want to stack weights up. Many beginners start with ring or fishing weights as it gives them more flexibility.

Clamping

Clamping is much simpler than extending or hanging, but, by extension, is also more limited in what it can achieve. The basic idea is a clamp or grip that can be placed around the base of your penis to trap more blood inside and really increase the girth of you penis.

It can also be used to help with lengthening exercises. The draw to the clamp is that there are many cheap devices you can use – and potentially even devices which aren't made specifically for clamping.

How it works

You can buy a purpose-built penis clamp for this, but many people use general purpose clamps. What you need is a device that will trap the flow of blood in your penis, more intensely than your hand alone can.

It works a bit like a super erection. The clamp stops blood leaving the penis, but blood can still enter, though to a limited degree, and this should allow it to expand the issue to a penis that is larger than it might normally be.

The expansion in penis tissue can then be lightly massaged (though you needn't do this) and over time will lead to a long term expanded penis. This is particularly good for girth and, in general, is unnecessary for length gains.

Using a clamp comes with a warning. It can be dangerous to build up this level of pressure in your penis, though not dramatically dangerous, and you leave yourself open to injuries like blisters.

It is recommended you don't start clamping until you have built your penis strength levels considerably and you only do it for at most twenty minutes a day. If the risk sounds like too much for you, then opting not to clamp at all is not a goal breaker. Gains can still be happily made without a clamp.

If you prefer kegels and extra use of hand-girth exercises can help you match the girth gains you get with clamping.

Step-by-step for safe usage

It is important that to do this safely you use lots of padding between the base of your penis and the grip. Placing a grip on your bare skin could lead to welts, blisters, and rashes. You should never be in any pain when doing this and you might want to consider using a timer to make sure you aren't clamping for too long.

You will need a level 4 or full erection to clamp properly, and you want to get hard first so there is more blood to trap in your penis. Lubrication is not necessarily required for this as you don't need to massage or exercise your penis to do this; however, lubrication can help many men achieve a stronger erection. Training yourself to get to this full state of arousal can be a useful exercise on its own.

One of the difficulties of clamping is that maintaining an erection, while sitting around doing nothing particularly erotic can be difficult. Make sure to have something stimulating at hand and to stop yourself getting too soft during the exercise. A clamp traps blood in, but since you won't have it on too strongly, it's possible that a loss of erection will stop the exercise.

1. Get your penis hard and then wrap your padding around the base of the penis as close to the pelvis as possible. You want thick padding here – a sock is about the level of thickness you will need.

2. Put the clamp around the part of your penis that has padding around it and then securely it firmly, but not tight enough that you are fully restricted yet.

3. Make sure your penis is at its full hardness and then slowly pull the clamp tighter, but loosen if you feel any pain or nipping. You need a clamp that can quickly be undone for this in case you do go too far.

4. Maintain this level of hardness and practice some kegels. Continue this for 5 to 10 minutes (stop if you start experiencing discomfort).

5. Take a break and rest your penis with a hot towel and then do another rep for a maximum of 20 minutes a day.

Consider taking a rest day or only doing 10 minutes some days so that you do not over-exercise your penis. A few light kegels should be enough, and you don't need to do any intense jelqing for a clamp to have an impact.

Take things slowly with clamping and ease into the level of clamping and pressure you induce. If you see any discoloration of the penis or it begins to feel cold or numb, then you are clamping too tightly and need to pause. Going too hard could cause longer term problems that run counter to your larger penis goals.

Many people like to make a choice between hanging, clamping, or extending and try not to do all three too frequently. If you are doing intense hanging sessions, consider avoiding clamping too long or too often at the same time.

Which device to buy

You have three options when trying to clamp. The first is the purpose-built devices such as the ThickerMan clamp. It's a padded clamp that comes with a large washer which is screwed in to create a tighter grip.

This device will certainly get the clamping job done, but some users claim it pinches a little too much and the device is more expensive than it needs to be.

By far the most popular product is simple cable clamps. They work a bit like a zip tie, but they aren't as constricting and you have more control of the tightness and how quickly they can be undone.

They will need considerably padding to be used comfortably, but padding is cheap and so are cable clamps. Be sure when buying clamps you do not get something like a zip tie which cannot be easily undone.

Practice using the device before trying it out on your penis.

The third option is to get a cock ring from an adult store or online. These are not as powerful as a clamp, but they can be used in effect with kegels and girth exercises to help boost your growth speed. You could also potentially use padding, like bandages, to create a lightly clam on their own.

Pressure Pumps

Pressure pumps, or penis pumps as they are better known, have been around for a long time and they are well-documented as cures for erectile dysfunction. Primarily they are used for larger erections or overcoming trouble getting an erection, but they can be used to help you get a larger penis.

These are sometimes overlooked by the penis enlargement community; because they can't be used with other exercises, and the industry has a habit of over engineering them to inflate the price. They are also not as effective in creating long term gains as an extender or a hanger. Some also argue that clamping or a cock ring can produce largely the same effect as a pump for far less money.

They work by creating a high-pressure seal around the length of your penis which will then cause it to enlarge in size, but only temporarily. This trapped blood, however, can then be used in penis growing exercises, and, over time, it should expand the tissue of the penis so that it can grow larger.

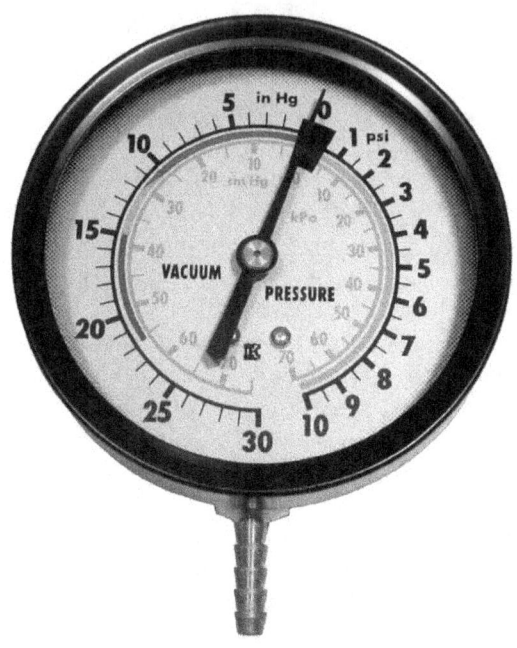

How does it work

There are two main types of penis pumps: air pumps and water based pumps. However, they all work to the same principle. You place a cylinder over your penis, which goes down to the base and creates a seal.

Pressure is created and a vacuum then makes the tissue of the penis expand to fill the space inside. Of course, too much pressure would make your penis explode and there's only so far it can expand. This means the size of the cylinder is limited and you have a pressure gauge to make sure you are staying safe.

Good quality pressure pumps should not allow you to create enough pressure to do any actual damage to your penis. They come with a release valve so that you can immediately put air back in and reduce the pressure. The worst that would happen is blistering o ruptured blood vessels, but these are by no means trivial injuries and should be avoided.

It is important that you pump slowly when using it, as small pumps can create large changes in pressure. Cheaper models made purely for getting erections may not come with a proper pressure gauge – so make so to shell out for that feature.

Both the air and the water pumps work in the same way by extracting air from a contained space to create a vacuum. For long term users the water option is often favored as it is slightly more comfortably, by many accounts.

The water model works by filling the cylinder with warm water, before placing your penis in and allowing some of the water to leave from the top valve. This creates a similar vacuum and it has the addition of being able to be used in the bath with no need for lube to create a better seal.

The pump can be used for 15 to 20 minutes a day for as long as you are happy to keep using it.

Step-by-step guide for safe usage

Using the pump should bring you to an erection, but if you want to save time you can get to a level 4 erection before using the device if you wish. It's best to sit down to use the device, and for a water pump a nice warm bath is the best place to use it.

Pubic hair may get in the way of making the seal and with the air models you may want to use lubricant to create a stronger seal. In the step-by-step guide we will be looking at a water pump, but they both operate in similar ways.

1. With the valve closed fill the cylinder of the pump with water and you can then place your penis inside the cylinder. Excess water will come out and you should have a strong seal made. You should not place your scrotum in the cylinder.

2. Once you have tilted and moved the pump so that you have a strong seal, you can open the valve end on the pump.

3. With most devices you can place both hands at the top of the cylinder (not covering the valve) and then pull down for a pump. This should be done slowly and the device should make it clear how much you need to do this to create a proper vacuum.

4. If the vacuum is too intense start again, but once you are at the right setting allow the pump to rest like this for 15 minutes. You may have to hold the pump to keep it in the right position. When you are finished simply release the valve.

Penis pumps are generally safe and easy to use, while giving you an immediately larger penis to enjoy, and then after a few months you should see longer term gains. The pump is an excellent way to warm-up for later exercise and can be used while bathing to cut down on work-out time.

Which device to buy

The main consideration is whether you want a water or air pump – water pumps are usually called, "hydro pumps" and air pumps are typically just sold as 'penis pumps'.

Some reviewers and users claim one is better for erectile dysfunction and the other better for penis growth. However, there is little evidence for this and they should have a similar impact on penis enlargement.

People like air pumps because they are often cheaper, they usually come with a pressure gauge, and you don't have to get wet or take a bath to use one.

The advantages of a hydro pump is that they are usually more comfortable thanks to the warm water and less pinching with the seal; in addition, they are designed so that only so much pressure can be made with them, meaning they are safer to use for many people.

The most popular hydro pumps are the Bathmate and the Hydro Max – which should equally serve you well. A good brand of air pump is the Squeeze Ball.

While the prices of some of these devices are quite high, you don't want to go for a cheap and poorly made device. A weak seal will mean you don't get much of a vacuum and an air device without a gauge can lead to over-pumping and too much pressure. As long you avoid the novelty penis pumps, nevertheless, you should be fine with the choice you make.

Which device to use

Choosing a device is largely up to what your goals and your personal preferences. If you don't want to use a device then gains are still perfectly possible.

If you are looking for length gains then the extender and hangers are the best option. If you are looking specifically for girth (and are not too concerned about length) then a clamp or pump will be the best option.

Extender and hangings devices come in at similar price tags, and since they operate in a largely similar fashion, they also have gains at a similar time frame. Extenders are easier to use, and can be in use while you perform other activities – however, you will need to use them for longer. Hangers require more advanced skills, but you only need to use them for a shorter period each day.

Clamps and pumps are both not as effective at enlarging your penis, as the other two devices, but they do form part of an essential penis enlargement regime. A clamp can be bought for a few dollars, whereas the pump may cost a few hundred in some instances.

The pump is quicker to use and more comfortable, but if you opt for a hydro pump you will only get to use them in the bath. For many people, an extender or Hanger, and a clamp should be enough to see very significant gains.

The surgical option

Surgery is often seen as a valid choice for many types of body modification, but it is not often turned to for penis enlargement by the community at large. This is because while there are methods to surgically lengthen the penis, many of them are extreme and don't actually make much more impressive gains than non-surgical options.

They also tend to be gruesome to think about and since not all plastic surgeons will do them, the price can go up considerably depending on your location.

There are two main types of surgery you can look at – one involves cutting part of your penis ligament so it will lean forward, and the other involves implanting various substances (silicone or fat for example) into your penis so it can increase in girth.

While the former option of cutting a ligament does work and is available at many practices, implants are used less often and have a tendency to not work as often as they do work.

For those struggling with erection a rod can be placed in your penis that can then be inflated to induce an erection. The rod will fractionally increase penis length, but it's not a true enlargement.

As you might deduce by the existence of this guide, implants and surgery in general are not popular and often fail to give people their desired results. However, many people are happy with the surgery they receive and it is possible to get it done at a respectable clinic with consistent results.

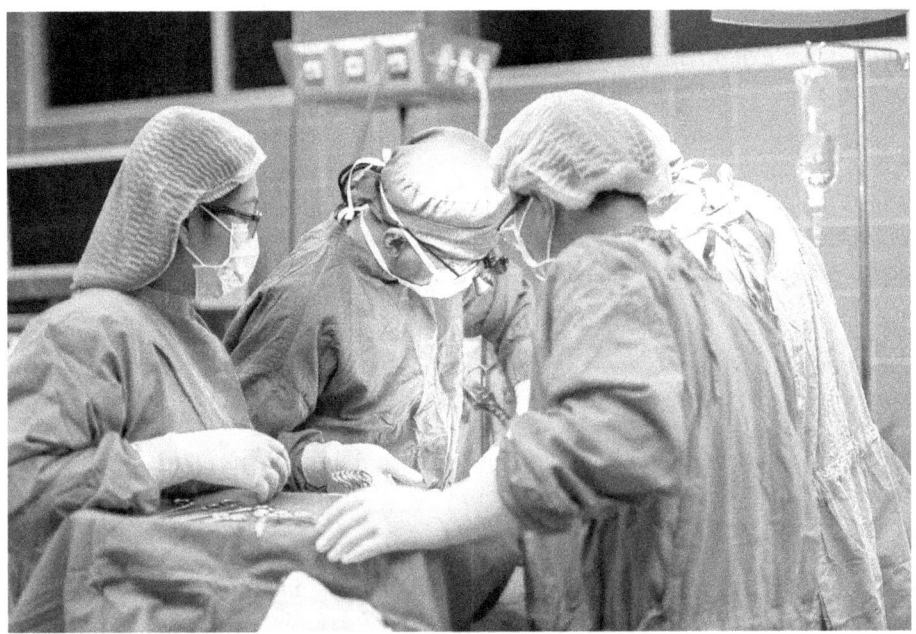

How surgery works

There are two main operations you can get done in a standard clinic in the West. The first is a lengthening surgery which works by cutting a ligament that runs from your penis up to your pubic bone.

This allows your penis to fall forward by as much as 2 inches – although technically no growth has occurred to the shaft of the penis. After this the ligament is reattached and healed up. This, however, only truly increased the length of your flaccid penis.

The second operation is to increase girth and this is done with liposuction. Fat is taken from your thigh and injected into the penis, which can increase girth by 2 inches as well.

Some surgeons will use a layer of skin tissue from elsewhere in the body in place of fat.

If you are interested in the surgical option then your healthcare professional will further explain the procedure and how it will work. They can both be done as outpatients and don't take more than a few hours to perform.

Is it worth it?

Prices vary but will start at a few thousand dollars and you do need to get the operation done by a professional. You can seriously damage your body if you try to get this done on the cheap.

So why doesn't everyone just have these operations done instead of doing year long penis workouts? Chiefly, people don't go through with it because the surgery doesn't really guarantee results.

How long your penis can be lengthened by cutting your penis ligaments depends a lot on your natural body shape. One study suggested the average growth was less than half an inch.

After surgery the penis will point further down and sometimes there will be scarring and sometimes the penis may look like it is coming out of the scrotum instead out of the abdomen.

The girth surgery can be even less effective, as your body naturally reabsorbs fat and as much as 90% of your gains can disappear within a year. The fat may also not distribute evenly along the shaft of the penis, and you can be left with a lumpy penis.

For these reasons, at its current state, penis enlargement surgery does not have much going for it. Your healthcare professional will be able to better inform you about the likely results and what you can expect if you are still interested.

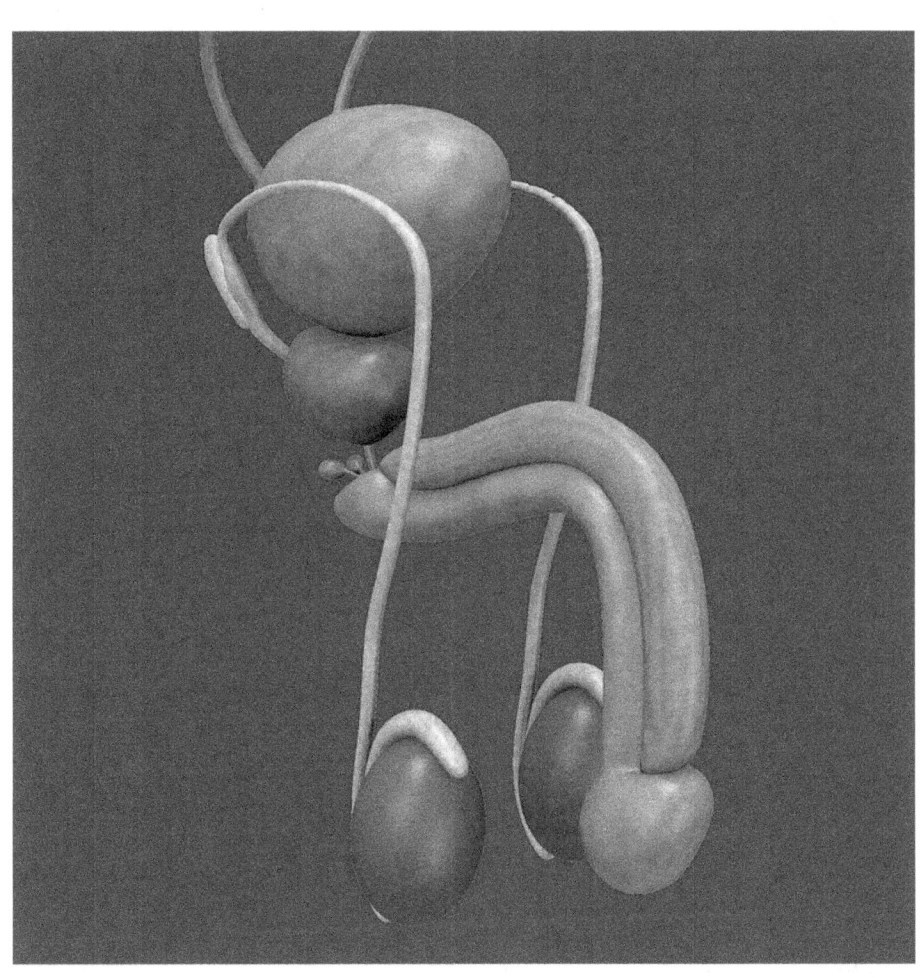

Penis workout regimes

Now we've gone through the many techniques, devices, and exercises you can do to get a longer penis, we're going to look at some potential regimes you could follow to start making gains yourself.

We'll look at the considerations you have to make beforehand and then run through the kind of day you can expect with different intensity regimes.

How to choose a regime

If you want a larger penis then it is going to take time, consistency, and real dedication. You cannot physically change your body with only a few weeks work – and it's important that you commit to a regime you can handle.

If you already have an average sized penis and you merely want a quick solution then shaving your pubic hair, working on foreplay, and a cock ring or penis pump might be more than enough to keep you happy. An optical illusion and a larger erection can have quite a large impact.

If you want a genuinely larger penis then you will need to commit for at least 6 months and potentially keep at some lighter exercises for years to come. No matter how intense or expensive you want to get, that level of commitment is necessary.

Intensity and expense are the next things to take into account. An hour a day should be enough to see changes and, in fact, six hour workouts every day will not yield you six times as quick gains. Using only the more gentle techniques will let you see changes, but they may not be as dramatic as if you had used a penis extender and done pelvis exercises.

How much you want to spend is up to you. You can make impressive gains for free, by just using hand techniques and choosing to have a longer warm-up instead of using supplements.

A year's supply of supplements and a good quality device could cost a considerable amount of money, but the effect of the supplements is quite strong and a device should be able to last for years.

If you are happy to spend any amount of money and you will do anything for a larger penis then surgery may be an option for you – however, don't build your expectations too high.

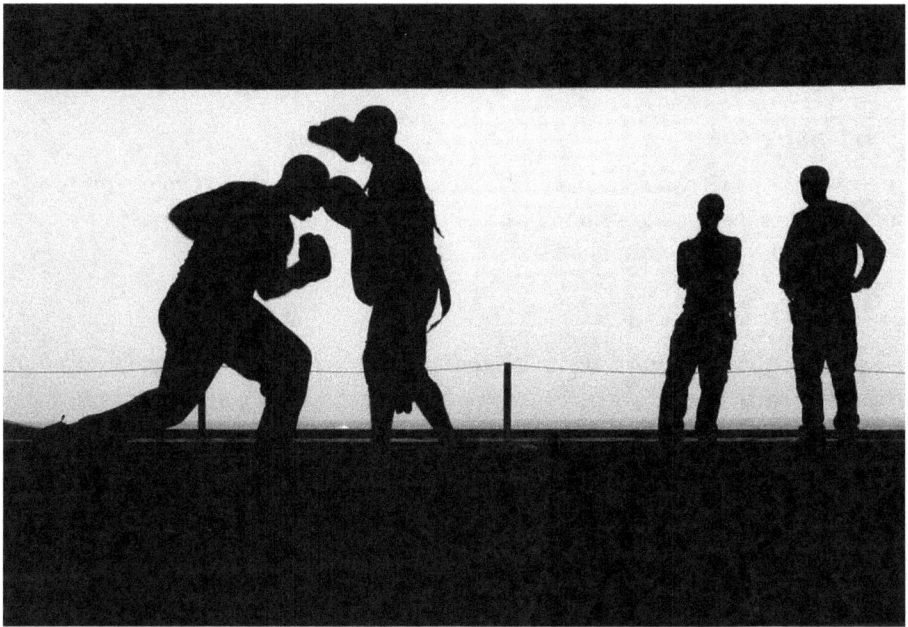

Creating a regime

If you want to create a regime for yourself then you should begin by trying out a few of the different techniques and seeing which works for you and which makes you the most comfortable.

Once you know that you need to consider your goals and what can get you there. Do you want a simply longer penis? A straighter penis? A penis with more girth? Or a fuller erection?

Longer penis

To increase the length of your penis you will want to carry out a significant amount of jelqs each day, as well as lots of warm-ups and basic stretches.

A penis extender or penis hanger is going to be the best options when it comes to devices, and a clamp can generally be helpful.

For a length based regime you want 70-80% of your workout to be focused on lengthening and you might want to consider allocating extra time simply for stretching or using a device.

Straighter penis

A straighter penis should come with a longer penis; however, if you want to focus on this specifically then try curve-correction jelqs and use a penis extender. These only need to be 50% of your regime.

More girth

Girth is all about getting more blood trapped in the penis so you can stretch out the inside of the penis. The girth exercises are a must, and you will want to use devices like the clamp and pressure pump.

For girth supplements can be especially helpful. If you are really interested in girth then as much as 60% of your regime can be based on girth building techniques – many will also help length so you needn't be too concerned about missing out.

Girth, however, is also a technique many will not feel a need to focus on too much and you can almost leave out specific girth exercises if you don't want to commit to too many devices or spread yourself too thinly.

Full erection

Many of the girth exercises will help with erections, but you to really give you a boost here supplements are essential, as are kegels. The clamp and penis pump will also help dramatically.

You won't need to dedicate more than 30% of your regime to erection strength, as some of the methods are more passive and you should generally have a stronger erection after working out more.

Other considerations

As well as working out your penis, you will also want to tone your body and increase your cardio fitness. This will help sexual performance, enhance your penis workout, and make your penis look longer in comparison to your sleek body.

It can be difficult to fit in everything though, especially if you are going to be spending two hours working on your penis each day. A good idea is to include natural exercise – such as running or walking to work, and to do pelvis strengthening exercises to get a double benefit.

Some penis stretches or even jelqing can be done while doing minor running exercises (though be very careful before you try this).

Kegels are something most men looking to increase their sexual performance should also consider. When working out your regime, include time for more passive activities like having your penis extender on and doing kegels. These can be fitted in around your basic workout time.

Sample regimes

Here we will look at some sample regimes you might want to adopt, or adapt, to your favored techniques or specific requirements.

As a primer for all of them you should be generally trying to get fitter and keeping a good diet. Getting plenty of protein and calcium is of course important, as is reducing the amount of salt, unhealthy fat and refined sugars in your diet.

Losing weight by lowering your calorie intake is one of the most effective ways of having a larger-looking penis. If you are particularly overweight you may want to look at what your real goals and priorities are here. Enlargement of your penis is not at all incompatible with weight loss, but it should certainly not replace it as a way of boosting your self-image.

Building muscles is not shown to have anywhere near the level of impact on perception of penis size as losing an overhanging gut will. This may seem like a huge demand on your time – however you are not looking for overnight results.

You need only get to a healthy weight and reduce too much flab around your thighs and belly. A relatively light cardio regime and some minor adjustments to your diet can have an enormous impact on this. The best regimes are always the ones you can see yourself sticking to longer term.

Whether you choose a free regime or not, supplements are recommended for all regimes as they provide a fantastic boost to growth and can be bought relatively inexpensively. Follow the instructions on your chosen supplement and make sure to use them when you are actively trying to increase penis length.

They increase growth and make the exercises you do even more powerful by allowing more blood in the penis and larger erections where they are required.

Each regime will be split into passive and active exercises. Passive activities are ones that you need to do each day, but they don't need to be figured into your allocated workout time. They can be done on the move, while watching television, or even at work in some instances.

Active exercises need to be part of your daily workout and need your full attention. If you only half do the techniques then you cannot expect to have full growth and, equally, you must commit to doing them properly. These regimes should not just be glorified masturbation sessions.

You do not necessarily need to do the exercises seven days a week, but you should do a minimum of 5 days a week, or limit yourself to 2 or 3 lighter days where you choose to be less intense with your exercises.

Your penis should be fatigued afterwards, but you should not experience a downturn in your sexual performance, skin disorders, or any significant pain or discomfort. If you do experience any of this then reduce the intensity of your regime immediately.

Free and easy regime

This is a regime that doesn't involve buying any devices and is aimed around helping beginners get started with penis enlargement. Nevertheless, it is also a regime that is good if you want a minimal and very achievable set of exercises to take up.

Many enlargers will want to use a regime like this, or a relaxed version of one, after they have gotten their desired gains and want to ensure they don't lose them.

It does not require any advanced skills and the risk of injury is low. You can expect to start noticing growth around the three month mark and if you remained dedicated this regime alone could see up to 2 inches of growth in a year's time.

2 inches may not sound like a lot on first hearing it, but, for the average man, that is over a 30% increase in the size of your penis and once you start getting much larger than 8 or 9 inches you are entering an impractical size for many women.

This regime is focused mostly on length, but should help with girth and sexual performance as well. Once you are happy with these exercises you can begin to increase the amount doing up to 1 hour of working out a day.

Passive exercises

Sit and stretch – 20 minutes – increases penis length and helps strengthen gains

Kegels – 100 reps – increases blood flow, erection strength, and pelvis muscles

Active exercises

Warm-up – 3 minutes – increases blood flow and flexibility

Basic penis stretch – 20 seconds in each direction

Simple jelq – 3 reps of 5 minutes – increases length and girth

Flaccid bend – 1 rep of 5 minutes – increases girth

Warm-down (repeat of warm-up) – 2 minutes

Free and intense regime

This is similar to the last regime but it is more intense and gives your penis a fuller workout. It remains free, and fairly simple, but you should see the most gains with this method, for the least amount of money.

Again it is a general purpose regime with a focus on length. You should try the less intense regime for the first few weeks at least so that you can discover your limits and how best to do the exercises.

Passive exercises

Sit and stretch – 20 minutes – increases penis length and helps strengthen gains

Kegels – 150 reps – increases blood flow, erection strength, and pelvis muscles

Steady tremble kegels – 50 reps

Active exercises

Warm-up – 3 minutes – increases blood flow and flexibility

Basic penis stretch – 20 seconds in each direction

Simple jelq – 3 reps of 5 minutes – increases length and girth

Flaccid bend – 2 reps of 5 minutes – increases girth

Twist and pull – 2 reps of 5 minutes – increases length

Towel deadlift – 1 rep of 5 minutes – increases erection strength and blood flow

Warm-down (repeat of warm-up) – 2 minutes

Strong all-purpose regime

This regime is one that uses either a hanger or an extender, which will increase gains by as much as 1 inch, and gives you a general increase in girth, length, and penis strength.

The regime is not particularly intense, but it will take more time and money than the free and easy regime. You needn't push it too far and start doing 6 hours of stretching a day; 1 or 2 hours is plenty of time to see gains and keep you disciplined enough to keep at it for a long period of time.

Passive exercises

Extender stretch – 1 or 2 hours – increases penis length and girth (optional: replace with hanging if you prefer)

Kegels – 100 reps – increases blood flow, erection strength, and pelvis muscles

Active exercises

Warm-up – 3 minutes – increases blood flow and flexibility

Basic penis stretch – 20 seconds in each direction

Simple jelq – 3 reps of 5 minutes – increases length and girth

Belt jelqing – 1 rep of 5 minutes – increases girth

Penis hanger – 2 reps of 10 minutes – increases length (optional: replace with extender if you prefer)

Warm-down (repeat of warm-up) – 2 minutes

Girth regime

If you really want to push getting extra girth in your penis then this is the regime for you. You will see some length gains, but this is all about pushing for girth and getting extra blood in your penis to keep that girth going.

It will require a clamp or pump, and you will need to practice kegels to start seeing a real impact and slowly build up to the amount recommended here - starting with as few as 50 or 100 a day.

You may want to try out a lengthening regime for a few months and then start focusing on girth. Alternatively, consider switching between girth and length from week to week.

Passive exercises

Kegels – 200 reps – increases blood flow, erection strength, and pelvis muscles

Steady tremble kegels – 50 reps

Active exercises

Warm-up – 3 minutes – increases blood flow and flexibility

Basic penis stretch – 20 seconds in each direction

Twist and pull – 2 reps of 5 minutes – increases girth

Belt jelqing – 2 reps of 5 minutes – increases girth

Clamping – 2 reps of 10 minutes – increases girth (optional: replace with pump if you prefer)

Penis pump – use for up to 30 minutes – increases girth (optional: replace with clamp if you prefer)

Warm-down (repeat of warm-up) – 2 minutes

Sexual enhancement regime

If you are looking specifically to improve your sexual performance, by being able to do more physically, then this is a sample regime you might like to follow.

This regime is all about getting a harder erection and being able to last longer, while getting in some smaller gains in length and girth. It's one of the easier and cheaper regimes to follow, but, of course, you won't have the same level of enlargement if you follow it.

Again, you can choose between the clamp and the pump here. The penis pump is arguably better in this capacity, as it can be used directly to improve the size and hardness of an erection.

Passive exercises

Kegels – 200 reps – increases blood flow, erection strength, and pelvis muscles

Steady tremble kegels – 50 reps

Active exercises

Warm-up – 3 minutes – increases blood flow and flexibility

Basic penis stretch – 20 seconds in each direction

Simple jelq – 2 reps of 5 minutes – increases girth

Belt jelqing – 2 reps of 5 minutes – increases girth

Clamping – 2 reps of 10 minutes – increases girth (optional: replace with pump if you prefer)

Penis pump – use for up to 30 minutes – increases girth (optional: replace with clamp if you prefer)

Warm-down (repeat of warm-up) – 2 minutes

All-out regime

This is the most complete and intense regime, and one that is only suitable for more experience enlargers. It requires a few devices and you will need to alternate between two different regimes and calculate rest days.

Hanging and clamping in particular require more resting as there is more room for injury – though advanced users should have more control over what they are doing at this point.

The passive exercises remain the same for both iterations of the regime, and you should do them even on resting days. This regime is intended to be done for shorter periods of time; for example, building you strength for 2 to 3 months with a simple regime, moving to the all-our regime for 6 months and then going back to a simple regime.

Passive exercises

Sit and stretch – 20 minutes – increases penis length and helps strengthen gains

Kegels – 200 reps – increases blood flow, erection strength, and pelvis muscles

Steady tremble kegels – 50 reps

Active exercises: Day A

Warm-up – 3 minutes – increases blood flow and flexibility

Basic penis stretch – 20 seconds in each direction

Twist and pull – 2 reps of 5 minutes – increases girth

Belt jelqing – 2 reps of 5 minutes – increases girth

Clamping – 2 reps of 10 minutes – increases girth (optional: replace with pump if you prefer)

Penis pump – use for up to 30 minutes – increases girth (optional: replace with clamp if you prefer)

Warm-down (repeat of warm-up) – 2 minutes

Active exercises: Day B

Warm-up – 3 minutes – increases blood flow and flexibility

Basic penis stretch – 20 seconds in each direction

Simple jelq – 3 reps of 5 minutes – increases length and girth

Belt jelqing – 1 rep of 5 minutes – increases girth

Penis hanger – 2 reps of 10 minutes – increases length (optional: replace with extender if you prefer)

Extender stretch – 1 or 2 hours – increases penis length and girth (optional: replace with hanging if you prefer)

Warm-down (repeat of warm-up) – 2 minutes

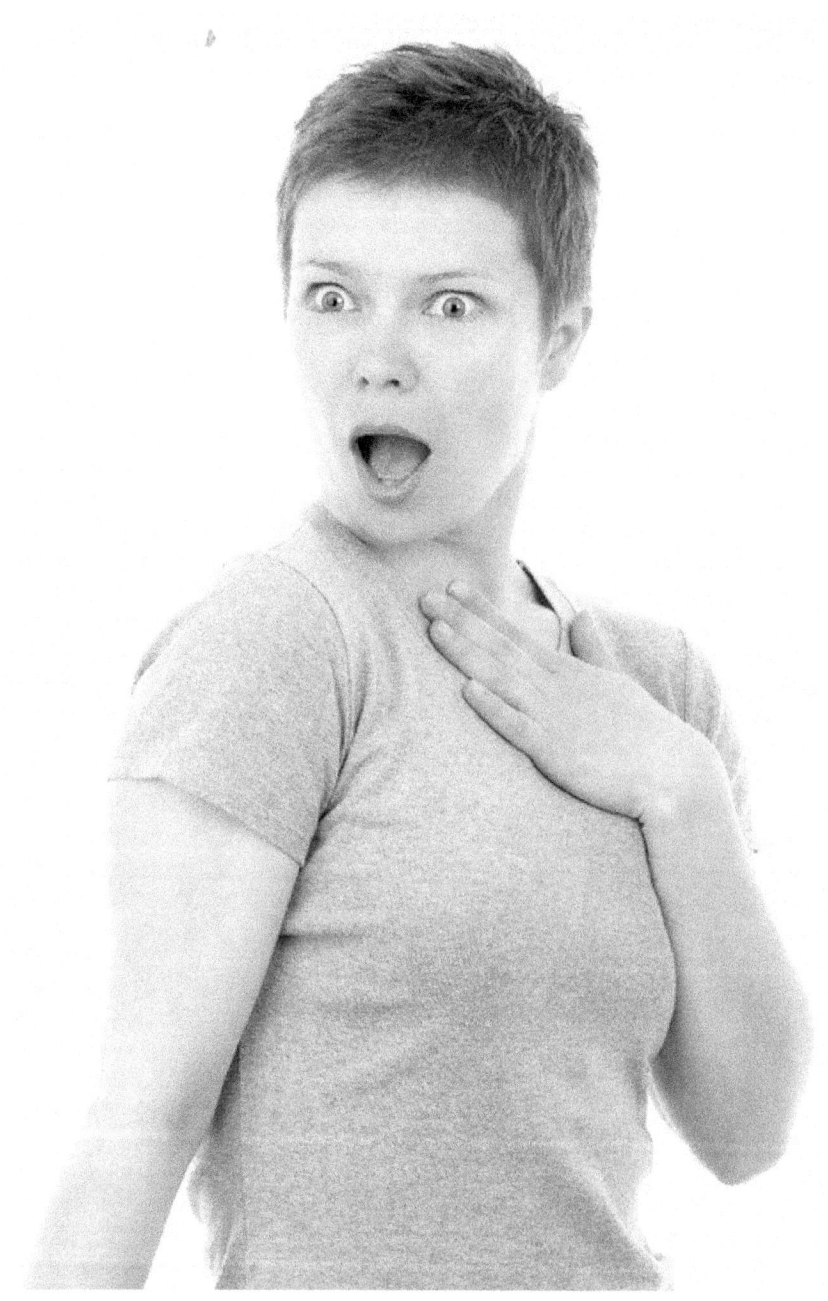

Conclusion

You now have all the skills you need to start making some truly impressive gains in penis size. If you've never undertaken a full scale body transformation or workout process like this, then you're in for an experience that can be truly life changing.

Many of us take a long time before coming to the decision to really commit to having a larger penis. It's sometimes hard to get past the social stigma attached to it, and we're often left feeling silly for wanting to improve ourselves in this way.

The truth is that having a penis that you feel is too small is a perfectly reasonable concern to have, and it's simply not worth worrying about such an issue if there is a solution available to you. And there is.

You've got the knowledge and the drive to make this happen – what's left now is ensuring that you get the gains you are after. Each person is different in the kind of results they can expect, and to really make these techniques work you'll have to exercise both patience and consistency.

The techniques are powerful, but they need to be executed properly and with strict discipline.

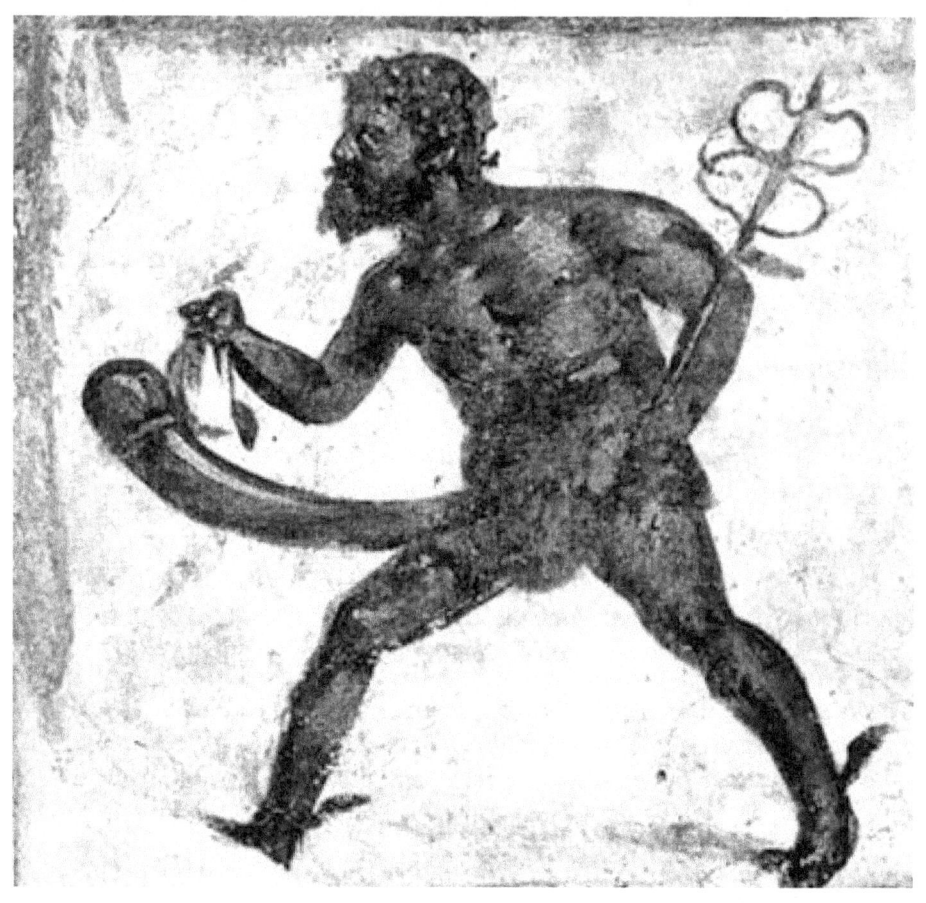

Patience

Once you've desired to work for a longer penis it can be a huge relief, but it can also leave you feeling that you've already lived too longer with your current penis size. You're excited about being able to have a larger penis.

However, patience is key to achieve true long term growth. This means you have to work through an initial awkwardness to make sure you are doing the techniques right, and to wait for change – and that may take at least two or three months before you can really get excited about your progress.

Not only does progress mean waiting for gains to happen – it also means not rushing ahead and pushing your body too far. The possibility of injury is real if you overdo things, and going too hard will not see you have a longer penis radically quicker. If you damage your body, then it will actually prolong your gains.

Consistence

Twinned with patience, is the need to be consistent in your exercises and techniques. You need to always be carrying out full techniques and not losing faith, or doing things in half measures.

Try to slowly increase intensity over time, and work to always be improving your technique – and not just trying to make them easier to carry out.

Build a regime that fits your needs and goals, keep working at making your gains and better understanding your body, and then you can have the ideal penis that you've always dreamed of.